KAREENA KAPOOR KHAN'S
PREGNANCY BIBLE

KAREENA KAPOOR KHAN'S PREGNANCY BIBLE

the ultimate manual for moms-to-be

with ADITI SHAH BHIMJYANI

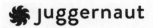

JUGGERNAUT BOOKS
C-I-128, First Floor, Sangam Vihar, Near Holi Chowk,
New Delhi 110080, India

First published by Juggernaut Books 2021

10 9 8 7 6 5 4 3 2 1

P-ISBN: 9789391165772
E-ISBN: 9789391165826

Typeset in Adobe Caslon Pro by R. Ajith Kumar, Noida

Printed at Thomson Press India Ltd

To the most handsome men in my life, my strength,
my world — Saifu, Taimur and Jeh

CONTENTS

FOREWORD

Dear friends,

Greetings and best wishes to all the beautiful mothers!

It gives me great pleasure to write this foreword as the 60th President of FOGSI. The Federation of Obstetric and Gyneacological Societies of India is a professional organization with 258 member societies and over 38,000 members spread over the length and breadth of the country. FOGSI is probably one of the largest membership-based organizations of specialized professionals.

> 'When you are a mother, you are never really alone in your thoughts. A mother always has to think twice, once for herself and once for her child.' Sophia Loren

It's not just the mom. An obstetrician too has to think and take care of two, the mother and the foetus. Every pregnancy is precious and should be a pleasant and memorable experience for the mother and her family. And our job as doctors is to ensure this. An obstetrician starts with preconceptional counselling and continues with regular antenatal care for the optimal outcome.

This book is the perfect companion for you on this journey and a useful supplement to your regular antenatal care. It tells you everything you need to know about your pregnancy, and we at FOGSI have vetted all the medical information for you.

I am delighted we were able to collaborate on this project this year as we have launched a campaign called 'FOGSI for all, always' to ensure that every Indian woman gets access to good gynaecological care. For to know and understand your body and the changes that take place in it is one step to becoming a healthier woman.

To this end, we have also started the DHEERA campaign to stop violence against women, as violence affects the mother's and baby's health during pregnancy. A healthy mother makes a happy family and a strong nation.

We wish you the best of health and happiness in your pregnancy.

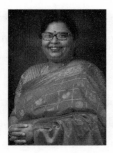

Dr S. Shantha Kumari

MD DNB, FICOG, FRCPI (Ireland), FRCOG (UK);
President, FOGSI, 2021–22; Professor, OBGYN; Chairperson, ICOG,
2018; Consultant, Yashoda Hospital, Hyderabad; Secretary, ICOG,
2015–17; Member, FIGO Committee for Human Rights, Refugees
and Violence Against Women, 2018–21; Vice President, FOGSI, 2013;
Managing Committee Member, IAGE; National Corresponding Editor,
JOGI; Organizing Secretary, AICOG, 2011; Chairperson, MNNRRC, 2008

INTRODUCTION

I am extremely passionate about whatever I do, whether it's getting in front of the camera, eating a 12-inch pepperoni pizza or writing this book. I do everything with determination and grit. I jumped at the idea of doing this book. I want you and every woman to know that things for me were just as normal (or difficult) as they are for you.

I had the same paranoias as every other mom-to-be, the same crazy symptoms, the same fears. And I also had the same excitement, the same wonder too. With this book I wanted you to be part of my journey and know that being pregnant is an amazing thing. And I also wanted to create a book that would give you the most authoritative and useful information not just about your trimesters but on issues such as postpartum depression, breastfeeding woes, nutrition, self-care and even on exactly what to shop for (I overdid it with Taimur!).

People think a celebrity pregnancy is super glamorous. And I did try and make it look like that when I was out and about! But I didn't feel that glamorous – who does when they are pregnant? I gained a lot of weight, got pregnancy spots and was ready to sleep by five every evening! Sounds familiar? In this book, I have been totally honest about everything I went through, from my crazy eating to fainting on a photo shoot out of exhaustion. I hope it will make you smile and comfort you too.

I decided when I got pregnant that I wouldn't hide anything. I was out there being as normal as I possibly could. And I wanted to bring that same spirit to this book. I am also super proud that I carried on my work right to the very end. Even though I have to admit I pushed myself too hard during Jeh's time.

The truth is I love being a mom. And I love acting. And I didn't want to give up on anything, even through my pregnancy. In fact after I got married, I did think hard about my decision to have a family. I thought people would see me differently.

But Saif told me I could do it all. He and I have worked hard to build a strong foundation for our relationship, and I truly believe my kids will always have that to stand on. And, hopefully, Jeh will be as confident as Taimur, because of his parents.

My mother-in-law was also among the first to tell me that I had to keep working. Her advice was to do whatever I wanted but with confidence. She did some great work in the movies after her marriage and kids and was a real inspiration. My mother is also a strong role model for me, and she and my father both told me I must keep at it. So I thought what the heck! I plunged headlong into not one but two pregnancies and I now have these two tots in my life who make every day feel a little crazy, a little special, a little exhausting, and a little rewarding.

And so here I am – writing these words, working, being a mommy, being active, being real. You know, my life often feels like the tree pose – where you're balancing on one leg. I think women do that beautifully.

I remember when I first held Taimur to my chest, properly, after the anaesthesia and grogginess had faded. My little boy became real to me that moment. The moment of birth I think for so many of us is too hazy. The reckoning comes later. As I held my little baby, smelling his infant smells, aware of how fragile and precious he was, I told myself I'd do it on my own, on my terms.

I set my own rules for Taimur, and those will apply for Jeh too. It was simple – to do the best I could and relax. I wasn't the most perfect mom the first time around. There is joy in messing up. I didn't know how to clean Taimur's poop or put on his diaper properly in the beginning. His pee leaked so often because his mother didn't secure his diaper perfectly. But here is some advice – mother to mother: it's about you and your comfort; do what is easy, do what works. When a mother is confident and comfortable, the baby senses it too.

It's why I returned to work so quickly. You've got to do what you've got to do. I knew I wanted to work till the day I popped and as soon as I could after. That being a mom was never going to be my only identity. Returning to work post-baby was heart-wrenching. I am sure that's the case with most mothers who get back to work. I remember leaving Taimur behind and going to night shoots with a crew of 150 people. I was so torn – trying to be professional on the shoot, while aching for my baby.

I have jumped back into my commitments soon after having Jeh too, though I definitely feel less rushed. It's normal to feel guilty. But trust me when I say Taimur doesn't love me any less today because I got my life back soon after I had him, and neither will Jeh. There is nothing like doing what you want to do. I will have one kid at my hand and another in my lap. I will be a mom and I will go back to work. I will rock all of it.

I am also so happy and grateful that I had my mother's help with Taimur. Yes, she is older now, which means Jeh is a challenge. She may be less hands-on, but she is a pair of reliable eyes for me, and I take much comfort in that.

We women place so much pressure on ourselves – we want to do it all. But everyone needs a little help. Take it. Hold that hand. Whether it's from family or household help. I would not have been half as functional without the help of my nurse who guided me through Taimur's time and is now with me for Jeh too. I am deeply grateful for both the women who helped me look after my babies and for the domestic staff who have looked after me and my family all these years. Saif and I are both working parents. Our lives would hardly be possible without them. And I want you to know that I don't have to be on Instagram putting a child to my breast to prove I am a hands-on mom. I just do the best I can, every single day.

You know, I was relaxed because I was prepared for both my kids and I had my rules in place. I am quite a freak when it comes to being organized! Of course, nothing fully prepares you for the actual birth and a live, kicking baby in your arms. There are so many unknowns. And there are so many things to which I still don't know how I will react. But that's what being a mom is. I always wanted kids. And I married the man I love. My kids are a symbol of my love, my life and my commitment. I may keep making mistakes. But I will power through.

Kareena Kapoor Khan

CONTRIBUTORS TO THE BOOK

This book was written consulting many medical and health experts, some of whom work with Kareena Kapoor Khan. We are extremely grateful for all their inputs.

Dr Mitossh Ruparel is a consultant radiologist with special interest in foetal medicine. He has over 20 years of experience. He has his specialty ultrasound clinic, Harmony Clinic, in Mumbai, where he connects expectant parents with their foetuses in a unique way.

Rujuta Diwekar is India's leading nutritionist and public health advocate. She is a vocal champion of using common sense and uncomplicating the act of eating right. Her books have sold more than 1.5 million copies and continue to define the discourse on food and exercise. She emphasizes a blend of traditional food wisdom and modern nutrition science for a healthy body and mind, best reflected through the mantra eat local, think global.

Namrata Purohit is the founder of the Pilates Studio and the Earth Circle. She is also an entrepreneur, author and an award-winning fitness instructor. She has been the youngest trained Pilates instructor in the world. She now runs studios across the country, training people from various fields including Bollywood celebrities, sports personalities and other fitness enthusiasts. She trains people at various fitness levels, working towards their goals and even specializes in pre- and postnatal Pilates, sports-specific training and injuries and special population.

Dr Rita Shah, a Lamaze consultant, is the director of Nine Months, a fitness and guidance programme for expectant mothers, established in 1990. She is a qualified Lamaze consultant, trained in prenatal and postnatal care from the United States and certified by ASPO Lamaze. She has prepared thousands of birthing couples all over the world to welcome their bundle of joy through live and online classes. She has been the head of the department of prenatal and postnatal care at Jaslok Hospital, Saifee Hospital and Leelavati Hospital in Mumbai.

Dr Neeru Vithalani, MD, DCH, is a consulting paediatrician, with over 40 years of experience. She is panel consultant at Breach Candy Hospital, Saifee Hospital, SRCC Children's Hospital and Bhatia Hospital in Mumbai.

Sonali Gupta is a clinical psychologist with 16 years of experience. Her counselling work is primarily focused on the intersection of grief, relationship dynamics, anxiety and compassion. She is a published author and columnist who is passionate about mental health advocacy. She has her own YouTube channel 'Mental Health with Sonali'.

Dr Ruma Satwik is a gynaecologist and infertility specialist at the Centre of IVF and Human Reproduction, Sir Gangaram Hospital in New Delhi. Apart from her clinical engagements, she is involved in infertility-related research and postgraduate and postdoctoral training programmes in her institute.

Dr Deepti Ghia, MD, DNB, FCPS, DDV, FIADVL (Phototherapy and Lasers), is a consultant dermatologist at Jaslok Hospital and All Doctors Clinic in Mumbai, and medical head at South Mumbai Dermatology. She was joint secretary of the Indian Association of Dermatologists in Maharashtra (2019–20).

Dr Prabha S. Chandra, MD, FRCPE, FRCPsych, FAMS, is a professor of psychiatry at the National Institute of Mental Health and Neurosciences (NIMHANS) in Bengaluru. She is in charge of the perinatal psychiatry service of NIMHANS, which is the first of its kind in South Asia. She is also president elect of the International Association for Women's Mental Health.

Dr Anahita D. Pandole, MD, DGO, DNB, FCPS, is a consulting obstetrician-gynaecologist and infertility specialist. She is panel consultant at Breach Candy Hospital and Jaslok Hospital in Mumbai.

Dr Vishal Sawant is a consulting psychiatrist and founder of Mindcare Institute, Mumbai.

Dr Rakhi Singh, MBBS, DGO, DRM, DPE, FICOG, FIAOG, is a leading senior fertility specialist with 25 years of experience and is director of Abalone Clinic in Noida. Her areas of interest are PCOS, infertility, obstetric care and endoscopy. She has also undergone advanced training in pelvic endoscopy and has been awarded a diploma in Reproductive Medicine and Embryology from Germany. She has authored and presented many research papers at national and international conferences and has written for *FOGSI Focus*, *Handbook of Drugs in Infertility* and *Jeffcoatte's Principles of Gynaecology*.

Dr Chandrika Anand, MBBS, MD, DNB, is the chief consultant of obstetrics and gynaecology at Fortis Hospitals and the founder–director of a PCOS centre in Bengaluru. She graduated from Kasturba Medical College with eight gold medals. With around 25 years of experience, she is committed to providing evidence-based quality healthcare to women of all age groups. Her areas of interest are high-risk pregnancies and PCOS. She has extensive experience managing PCOS and has created awareness amongst thousands of college students.

Dr M. Krishna Kumari is an obstetrician and gynaecologist with over 30 years of experience. She works as a professor in Apollo Medical College and as senior consultant at Medicover Hospitals in Hyderabad. Her special interests are high-risk pregnancies and critical care.

PART I

YOUR 40 WEEKS

My pregnancies

A celebrity pregnancy may appear very glamorous. You've seen me or other actresses in beautiful clothes, professional make-up, posing for magazines with our hair perfectly done, smiling and happy. Maybe you thought to yourself, damn, she is having such an easy pregnancy! But trust me when I say I am as normal as the next person. Whether it is morning sickness or exhaustion, crazy food cravings or the anxiety new moms feel, I have been through it, just like you.

My two pregnancies have been completely different – Taimur's pregnancy was like a movie, the whole thing was a dream. Reality hit during Jeh's pregnancy, which was much, much harder. However, I have approached both my pregnancies casually and done everything I wanted to do – from working to taking holidays to doing a photo shoot for this book just as I approached my due date! If there is one thing both the pregnancies have had in common, it's my determination that I wouldn't let it affect my day-to-day life.

I always knew I wanted to be a mother but I have never been bothered by the proverbial 'biological clock'. Saif and I had been married four years when I got pregnant at the age of thirty-six. We always talked about having children, but we never really actively tried, waiting instead for things to happen naturally in their own course.

I was on a lovely beach holiday in Koh Samui around the end of April 2016. Usually I adore the beach, relaxing by the sea with a glass of wine, and partying at night. But I felt unwell quite suddenly. It was a dull, nagging headache that just wouldn't go away. I thought perhaps it was the sun, so I stayed indoors. I even skipped a dinner party one night, which is very unlike me. I love parties!

Luckily I felt better at the end of the holiday and managed to pull through the flight, but when I got back home, the headache returned with a vengeance. It felt like a bad case of migraine. I never get headaches and so I called my doctor. He prescribed a spot of rest and Crocin, but also asked me if I could be pregnant and suggested I take a test.

When the test was positive, Saif and I were over the moon. It was something both of us had been looking forward to and it had happened so naturally, just like it was meant to be. We were overwhelmed.

Most people would say things like, 'Fab, wow, but you know your life is going to change.' In many cases women who are in the public arena tend to go into hiding during their pregnancy. This is especially true of actresses. It could be because of the weight gain, their health, or maybe wanting privacy during this moment. I approached my first pregnancy differently and took it head-on. Yes, 40 weeks from now there was going to be another person and my life was going to change, but I wanted to enjoy this moment. People love doling out advice any chance they get, but I told myself that I would do this my way!

Nor did I especially prepare. I did not read any pregnancy book, just the odd article online. I let my brilliant obstetrician-gynaecologist Dr Feroze Soonawala and nutritionist Rujuta Diwekar guide me through the rest. In case you haven't already figured it out, I have never done anything by the book! I was the most comfortable going to Dr Mitossh Ruparel for my ultrasounds – I didn't miss a single one!

Luckily, my first pregnancy was amazing. Taimur never troubled me in my tummy, although he troubles me now. I didn't have morning sickness, though I did get a little tired. Those headaches also stopped within the first two months.

I was energetic, and so very happy. I travelled for a large chunk of my pregnancy. We spent the better part of the monsoon at Saif's ancestral home in Pataudi. One major highlight was going to Rome. We stood in the Sistine Chapel with crowds of people, just Saif and I, in awe of the beautiful frescos up above us. We went to every site, every museum in Rome and Florence. Saif has been an art history student so travelling with him is like a lesson in itself! I partied like crazy too, often going to bed at 3 a.m. It was an amazing holiday – a lot of our close friends and even Saif's daughter Sara joined us at some point in the break. And of course I worked through my pregnancy and finished all my film and brand commitments. In fact, I was on my feet till a day before I delivered Taimur in December 2016.

But my experience during my second pregnancy was the opposite. It's not just me. Many women have drastically different experiences across their pregnancies – everything, from symptoms to cravings, can be poles apart. Maybe it had something to do with my age. I was pregnant with Taimur at 36 and at 40 with Jeh.

I found out I was pregnant with Jeh in May 2020, right in the middle of the global Covid pandemic and India's lockdown. We were all at home in Mumbai, with nowhere to go, feeling a little bit restless and hot, watching the headlines. That summer I got ill for four days – it was sudden, terrible nausea. I instantly knew I was pregnant.

We were all thrilled when my test was positive. This pregnancy was worrisome though. I was much less active. And I had an overriding sense of anxiety because of Covid, which I know a million others felt too. But, above all, I was just very sick. I was ridden with exhaustion and low blood pressure pretty much through my whole pregnancy and I had terrible nausea which stretched into the second trimester.

The first three months were especially bad. I was on nausea medication through the whole trimester. I was extremely tired and slept for 15–16 hours a day. I literally couldn't get my head up from the pillow! I couldn't eat. I would call my doctor desperately and beg him for any medicine that would make it all stop. I lost three kilos.

I could write a book on morning sickness! You know that constant feeling of being on the brink of nausea (like acid reflux combined with the urge to vomit)? I had that every single day for the first 17–18 weeks. On some days, the anti-nausea medication wouldn't even work. You wouldn't have wanted to meet me during that time – I was ratty, snappy and constantly belching. I would belch sitting on the sofa in the afternoon even without having had a heavy meal. Let me tell you there is very little glamour in a belching film star!

My doctor assured me that what I was going through was perfectly normal – that the first 18 to 20 weeks is when the baby is forming, which means my hormones were working overtime and racing against each other. My family and friends were full of sympathy.

They would keep saying, don't worry, this will pass. When you feel exhausted and ready to throw up all the time, you really don't want to hear all that. You just want to feel better! To add to all this was the extra pandemic-occasioned precaution. Touch wood, I had no scares, although Covid was a constant worry.

It all came as such a rude shock because I had expected this pregnancy to be exactly like the first one. Anyhow, I toughened up and decided to get on with it. If I was feeling very ill, I would take a day off and put my feet up but otherwise I remained active. I even shot a film (*Laal Singh Chaddha*) with Aamir Khan in Delhi, at the height of Covid, in my second trimester.

I was grateful that Saif, Taimur and I got to spend some time together when I was shooting in Delhi though. We moved to Pataudi and made that our base for a while. I commuted between Delhi and Pataudi every day. We often filmed at night – 7 p.m. to 7 a.m. – in Delhi. At the end of a gruelling day, I would collapse on to my bed, totally exhausted. I was determined not to moan about it and no one on the set knew what I went through.

Everyone around me – Saif, my friends, family, people on set – was paranoid about my safety. I took heart in the fact that hundreds of women like me continued to work through this scary and unpredictable time. It was my husband's unwavering support that sharpened my will. He would always say, 'Be careful, stay safe, you're a strong woman. If you want to do this, you can.' Without Saif and Taimur, I may not have survived the awful nausea and the lockdown stress. On an especially tiring day, I always had my mischievous little boy to make me smile and my husband to de-stress me.

Anyway, I finished all my brand commitments. I masked up and went out, ran the home, looked after Taimur and I even started on this book. I know how hard it is for pregnant moms with toddlers, having to manage a little daredevil along with your symptoms. I have been there!

On top of all this, we moved home less than a month before I delivered. Moving home is considered one of the most stressful things for a person, and here I was pregnant, sick and on my feet for 11 hours a day in my eighth month supervising the work. Insane? Well, Saif, Taimur and I wanted to be settled in our new home before the baby arrived, so I pushed it through. Carpenters, contractors, upholstery, kitchen: I did it all, despite the fear of Covid. Saif was away for work, and I know that it meant a lot to him that I managed this difficult time single-handedly. But it was our family home, and I can proudly say that my blood and sweat is in it.

There were good moments too! I managed to fit in a holiday and had a wonderful and relaxing break in Dharamshala with Taimur as Saif was shooting there for two months. The clean mountain air and fresh food really did wonders for me. We got to spend a lot of time together there. Himachal Pradesh is just beautiful, and the weather was perfect. We went on long walks, checked out the local food and enjoyed the green open spaces – especially Taimur. Besides Dharamshala, we also ended up in Palampur for a bit while Saif was shooting there.

I must take a moment here to add that by my eighth month, my exhaustion was next level. I had to slow down. I tried to fulfil a commitment I had made to a fashion magazine for a photo shoot but I got dizzy on set and had to be carried back to my vanity van. I felt like I was on the verge of collapse. Yet I couldn't help feeling extremely upset that I had failed to keep up. It had *never* happened to me before.

Now you really don't have to go as far as me. Work does make me feel happier, and I like pushing myself. I also credit my ob-gyn for giving me the confidence to work. Dr Feroze tackles every pregnancy differently, which is what I really like about him. He has delivered all the kids in mine and Saif's family. I myself was delivered by his father, Dr Rustom Soonawala.

Throughout my second pregnancy, Dr Feroze always maintained that he wanted me to be safe but he did not want to stop me from doing anything. He said, 'Mask up, wash your hands, maintain social distance and stay in a bubble as much as you can.' That's it.

Let's face it, vaccine or no vaccine, masks and social distancing will be a way of life for a few more years. I didn't want to miss out on anything because I was pregnant. And this difficult pregnancy taught me so much of what I was capable of. I began the journey with anxiety and sickness – but I ended it feeling a tremendous satisfaction that I had been able to achieve everything I set out to.

1

YOUR FIRST TRIMESTER

In Taimur's time, when my pregnancy test was positive, Saif and I were thrilled. We knew we wanted to be parents but had never thought about when it would be. We actually never expected to get pregnant; we weren't actively planning a baby. But we were very happy, as were our families. I was also nervous. And that tremendous feeling of joy (and anxiety) didn't change when I found out I was pregnant with Jeh. Nor was I any less excited than I was the first time.

Congratulations! Your pregnancy test result shows two pink lines. You may also have done the follow-up hCG blood/urine test by now to confirm your pregnancy (see box 'What is hCG?').

Your pregnancy is divided into three trimesters. Your first trimester covers the first three months of your pregnancy, or about 12 to 13 weeks (starting from the first day of your last menstrual cycle). A pregnancy is calculated to last 40 weeks, though not everyone always reaches week 40. When you divide 40 weeks by three trimesters, you get roughly 13 weeks per trimester.

WHAT IS hCG?

Human chorionic gonadotropin (hCG) is a hormone produced during pregnancy and it is detectable in your blood and urine. Home pregnancy tests work by detecting hCG in the urine while the pregnancy confirmation blood test checks for hCG levels in the blood. Small levels of hCG can be detected even from eight days after ovulation. It rises rapidly during the first few weeks, doubling and quadrupling its levels every few days. A growing hCG level is a sign of a healthy pregnancy in the very early weeks. Your doctor may ask you to take a blood test to check its rise after you first test positive. In some cases, such as for IVF pregnancies, you may need to take up to three hCG blood tests over a 10-day period to check if it's rising as this indicates a healthy pregnancy.

The first two weeks of what you call your pregnancy is actually the pre-conception stage when your body is getting ready – your uterus is thickening and you're ovulating. After this, when the sperm makes its way to the egg, which is waiting in the fallopian tubes, you're about to conceive.

When fertilization happens within a day of ovulation and the sperm and egg unite, a little embryo is formed which immediately starts making its way to your uterus. The embryo's cells are dividing all the while to eventually form your baby. This goes on through the first four weeks.

Week four till the end of trimester one is when the real action starts. This is a tremendously exciting phase when your baby goes from a single cell to an embryo to becoming a tiny human-shaped being, with fingers and toes, skin and hair, functioning organs and a beating heart.

Usually **it is from week 5 to week 13 that most of you will feel the onslaught of a variety of pregnancy-induced symptoms** like headaches, spotting, mood swings, tender breasts, morning sickness, exhaustion/excessive sleep, sensitivity to smells and increased frequency of urination. Most miscarriages also tend to happen in the first trimester. The risk of a miscarriage drops sharply post the first 12 weeks of pregnancy.

Your body is going through huge changes during this time. Your hormones begin to go into overdrive, trying to make this baby and to prepare your body for a pregnancy. Through this time, you will feel a range of emotions. Immense happiness and excitement at the prospect of parenthood and anxiety about the impending nine months, birthing, breastfeeding and being a mom, especially if this is the first time for you. Not much will be evident from the outside though. Most women barely see a change in weight or appearance in trimester one. A few women even lose some weight owing to a decrease in appetite or morning sickness. The baby bump isn't visible either.

DATING MY PREGNANCY

You'll hear the terms LMP and EDD very often in the early stage of your pregnancy. Your EDD is the Expected Delivery Date, which will be determined via ultrasounds and by calculating 40 weeks forward from the first day of your last period, also known as Last Menstrual Period (LMP). Most women do not deliver on the exact EDD. Your LMP is an important date for you to bear in mind. If you don't remember your LMP, which is also quite likely to happen to many of us, your early ultrasounds will approximate your pregnancy dating based on the yolk sac and other measurements.

In your first trimester, you'll begin your first prenatal visits to the doctor and your first ultrasounds which will assess the viability of your pregnancy, measure your foetus and give you near-accurate dates of delivery (see box 'Dating my pregnancy').

A look at the first trimester for an IVF mom

Your IVF cycles have assisted you with the implantation of the embryo. Once that is complete and you're pregnant, your baby will grow in the same way as a baby conceived naturally, and you will feel the same as any would-be mom. There are a few differences. You will be given some additional medication in the first trimester such as progesterone (which also may sometimes be given to moms who have conceived naturally), you'll have more ultrasounds and you may conceive multiples. However, most IVF labs today strive to achieve a single healthy pregnancy by implanting a single embryo. Triplets are a rarity in the current practice, even with IVF.

Timeline: You will be pregnant about two weeks after your embryo transfer. You will be asked to do an hCG blood test 14 days after the embryo transfer. This blood test will confirm your rising hCG levels. An initial ultrasound will be conducted to make sure everything is going well: to check the yolk sac, to check how many embryos are growing and to see whether they're growing in the right place, which is your uterus. If all is well, a second ultrasound will be scheduled for a few weeks later. Women with high-risk/precious pregnancies or multiple embryos may be asked to follow up with repeat ultrasounds (see box 'What Is a Precious Pregnancy?'). Once you're in the clear with both these ultrasounds, you will breathe a lot easier.

Care: You will be put on folic acid and a progesterone hormone support regimen. You will be under the care of your fertility doctor in the early stages of pregnancy. After a successful conception (post seven to nine weeks), you may (or may not) move from your fertility specialist to the care of another obstetrician-gynaecologist (also referred to as an ob-gyn) who will deliver your baby. There are many ob-gyns who are fertility specialists and will see you through till the end of term – from your IVF cycle till the birth of your baby. Your medical protocol will not differ. On an average, moms of IVF babies face longer spells of first trimester bleeding or spotting which might end up with them being put on bed rest. Don't hesitate to seek your doctor's advice for everything: for exercise, yoga, travel and safe sex.

What's happening to your body in the first trimester?

In my first pregnancy, my first trimester symptom was a headache for just four days. The second time around, I was nauseous for nearly 18 weeks and exhausted till the very end of term. Every pregnancy is different, even if it is the same mom!

While your baby bump isn't going to show this early, your reproductive organs are working overtime right now. As we just read, the first three weeks of your pregnancy is when your body is setting the stage for you to conceive. Light spotting is very common around the time you would generally get your period, because the fertilized egg is attaching itself to your uterus lining. The first and most distinct sign of pregnancy is amenorrhea, which is the scientific term for absence of menstruation.

It is at **week 4** that the zygote starts burrowing into your uterine lining in what is called the implantation phase. What starts as a cluster of cells in your uterus grows into an embryo which is the size of a tiny seed. This little embryo is encased by an amniotic sac. Your placenta is developing and creating a ton of hCG right now.

At week 5 you might perhaps feel the first hints of pregnancy symptoms, like morning sickness or fatigue (if they haven't set in already). Until this stage, your baby has been receiving most of its nourishment from your uterine wall.

You may experience your first hint of food cravings at **week 6**. This sesame seed–sized embryo now sprouts into a tadpole-sized embryo. The hormones in your body – chiefly progesterone and oestrogen, the two main pregnancy hormones – go into overdrive to create an environment that is conducive to the growth of your baby. At the same time, the internal genetic code and epigenetic variations of the embryo are working to develop your baby too.

By **week 7**, the crazy hormone influx and fluctuating blood volume is very likely to induce a whole host of symptoms, from nausea, exhaustion and sleepiness to tender breasts, headaches, vomiting and mood swings. Now is when you start getting careful with your nutrition – after all, your baby's brain is developing at this very moment, apart from pretty much all its organs.

At **week 8**, your slowly growing uterus (and hormones, of course!) can generate some lower back pain. Ease into your exercise routine and stretches (with guidance and with your doctor's approval), if you haven't done so already.

By **week 9**, your pregnancy symptoms may still be on the rise or may have stabilized. Keep up the blood circulation by staying active. It is quite normal to feel nervous and also to overanalyse your symptoms. Be vigilant for any red flags and stay in touch with your doctor (see section 'How will I feel: Symptoms of trimester one').

By **week 10**, as your uterus grows and your body is processing your pregnancy, your kidneys work overtime. You may feel the need to urinate more frequently. This is because for the first 12 to 13 weeks, your growing uterus is low in your pelvis, thereby pressuring your bladder. But that doesn't mean you should stop drinking water. Your body is also producing more oestrogen than it ever will in your entire non-pregnant life. Your oestrogen and progesterone levels stay high till the end of your pregnancy. Your high hCG levels begin to even out from your second trimester.

Week 11 will continue in the same manner. What are these crazy hormones doing for you though? They're relaxing your muscles, preventing uterine contractions, maintaining your endometrial lining and increasing blood flow to nourish the baby.

Congratulations! You're pretty much at the home stretch of your first trimester at **week 12**. Your chances of miscarriage will now be lower. For some of you, the pregnancy symptoms will begin to ease out as you hit **week 13**.

What's your baby up to?

Saif and I loved going for our scans together. He accompanied me for several scans during Taimur's time. Though I have to say I often went by myself too. I chose to do almost all my scans in 3D/4D. I loved my ultrasound sessions and would be totally engrossed by the scans as my sonologist ran me through every detail of the baby's development. During Jeh's time, we were at the height of Covid, and I was more cautious about leaving the house. While I didn't miss any of the important scans, I was in and out of the clinic more quickly. And I most often chose to go alone.

A QUICK END-OF-MONTH SUMMARY

Month 1
What's forming? The amniotic sac and placenta to keep the foetus safe; a rudimentary face; circles for eyes; throat, mouth, jaw, blood cells
What's the size? 0.25 inch
What's the shape? Grain of rice
What's the weight? Difficult to gauge

Month 2
What's forming? Facial features like eyes; buds that will soon become arms, legs and ears, ending in fingers and toes; neural tube (that eventually forms the brain, spine and central nervous system); digestive tract; bones
What's the size? 1–1.5 inches
What's the shape? Tiny tadpole
What's the weight? 9.45 grams

Month 3
What's forming? Arms, fist, fingers, fingernails; legs, feet, toes, toenails; the start of teeth; reproductive organs; urinary and circulatory systems; a functional liver
What's the size? 3 inches
What's the shape? Pea pod–sized human
What's the weight? 28–29 grams

Week 1: This starts from the first day of your last menstrual cycle. So you're not quite pregnant yet. Your body is still preparing for the possibility of a pregnancy, which basically means your uterus lining is thickening.

Week 2: You're ovulating and at your most fertile. The eggs in your fallopian tubes are ready and waiting for sperm. This is when you conceive.

Week 3: The sperm and egg have become a zygote. It's a single cell, indulging in a lot of activity. The fertilized egg is making its way to attach itself to your uterine wall. All the while, its cells are dividing copiously (cells that will later form the baby's organs and body) and the chromosomes from the sperm and egg are gelling together.

Week 4: The embryo is in your uterus and beginning to get protection from the amniotic sac. The attached yolk sac and your placenta are nourishing your baby at this point of time. The embryo looks like a grain of rice. It is good to keep in mind that the all-important 'neural tube' is forming in your embryo approximately between day 17 and day 30. The brain, spine, skull and spinal cord develop from this neural tube.

Week 5: The foetus actually develops rapidly from day 31 of your pregnancy. What looks like a series of little tubes and layers starts forming into the baby's important organs. The neural tube is closing. It is at this stage that a growing foetus can develop neural tube defects.

Week 6: The heart begins to form and starts to beat – at 160 to 180 beats per minute, which is pretty fast (FYI, yours is 60 to 100). You'll see it in your ultrasound! Your baby looks like a

C-shaped tadpole and is now growing bones. The lungs, eyes (like two little black dots, which cannot see yet) and basic digestive system are emerging. The brain is actually beginning to form now into distinct areas with a bundle of nerves within.

Week 7: What's amazing is that pretty much every organ of your baby has begun to form (heart, kidneys, liver, lungs and intestines). His limbs have just sprouted (like little flat buds), soon to become hands and feet. The all-important umbilical cord is now nourishing your baby with oxygen and nutrients. Your baby's main eye parts (cornea, iris, pupil, lens and retina, all of which enable vision) start developing from now. In the second month, your baby begins to move, though there is no way for a mother to feel that. The little one is growing about 1 mm a day! The right and left hemispheres of the baby's brain are forming.

Week 8: Your baby looks like a kidney bean and is just about developing his face and a hint of a nose, ears, upper lip and eyes. You'll see two little depressions that are soon to become nostrils. The C-shaped curve slowly begins to straighten. It may sound unbelievable, but his little cartilages (later to be bones) are already strengthening, and the cerebral cortex is forming. And even more amazing is that your baby's heart is beating twice as fast as yours: 150 times per minute.

Week 9: His body is way bigger than his head, but the tadpole tail slowly turns into two legs. Your baby is building muscle. The sex organs and reproductive system begin to take shape from here. He is the size of an olive. His jaws open and close from now on, so your baby is yawning away.

Week 10: Your baby has teeny little elbows that can already bend; mouth and ears; a clearly visible umbilical cord; and a brain that's forming connections and growing bigger – it's actually working by now. He has wide-open eyes but no vision. The little fingers are more open now than later on in your pregnancy, when your baby will have balled-up fists. The true miracle is that his vocal cords are developing. Another 30 weeks, and your baby is going to be using these on you.

Week 11: Your baby is sized like a two-inch prune. His eyelids have formed by now. His external genitalia are developing (your baby's genitalia cannot be clearly seen in an ultrasound till at least five more weeks post trimester one).* Your baby has still got a lot more head than body. Now there are fingers and toes on the hands and feet!

Week 12: Around this time, your baby's eyelids fuse shut and only reopen around week 28. The tiny body starts to even out with his gigantic head and begins to look more and more like a 'baby'. The kidneys begin to work by now, which means your baby's body is able to process amniotic fluid and produce urine. Yes, your baby is peeing! The muscles in his digestive tract are already contracting. He can kick a bit and curl his toes. And you know those lines and creases on your palms? They're called palmar flexion creases and they develop at 12 weeks in vitro!

Week 13: Growth is quick and more proportional. If you pick up a scale towards the fag end of your first trimester, your baby is three inches long and 28 to 29 grams in weight.

---

*It is illegal in India to use any technique to identify the sex of the foetus. In 1994, the Parliament of India enacted the Pre-Conception and Prenatal Diagnostic Techniques (PCPNDT) Act, also known as the Prohibition of Sex Selection Act.

Doctors in India are legally and morally bound to not reveal foetal gender.

(With inputs from Dr Mitossh Ruparel)

How will I feel: Symptoms of trimester one

I had very different symptoms during both my pregnancies. In Taimur's time, I had a short-lived spell of tiredness and headache. With Jeh, I was utterly exhausted for a large part of the nine months and severely nauseous for over four of them. Morning sickness, let me tell you, can last through the day!

Nausea, with or without any vomiting, is the most prominent symptom of your first trimester. What is called morning sickness can last all day and even carry on way longer than your first 12 weeks. A niggling headache, backache, sleepiness and tiredness are common, thanks to hormonal changes combined with fluctuating blood volumes. Your breasts may feel tender (but any anomalies – inverted nipples, sores, discharge or pain – need to be checked out ASAP).

Stay prepared for **hot flashes, dizziness, decreased (or increased) sex drive, changing vision** and an **increased frequency in urination**. Certain tastes and smells can really put you off. **Gum inflammation and gum bleeds** happen because of rising oestrogen levels. You can blame your hormones for pretty much everything!

You might suffer from **mood swings** and **emotional sensitivity** along with some food cravings. Why does this happen? Again, it's the two big hormones at play: oestrogen and progesterone. Oestrogen plays with your mood (so it can make you depressed, anxious or irritable) and progesterone works on relaxing your joints and muscles (making you feel tired and perhaps even sad).

Combine this with the anxiety of becoming a parent soon and potentially sleepless nights, and you may just become a cocktail of emotional volatility. Through the nausea and the emotions, take it easy and be kind to yourself. There is little you can do to alleviate the feelings.

A significant bout of morning sickness accompanied by vomiting and acid reflux might even cause some erosion of the enamel of your teeth. In some cases, you may already start to see a **slight swelling in your limbs** (feet and ankles mainly), although this is more likely to happen in later stages. Keep an eye out for excessive swelling as it could possibly be indicative of high blood pressure (BP). It is essential to keep track of your BP and your blood sugar because high BP can develop into pre-eclampsia (dangerously high BP) later on in pregnancy, and sugar levels can elevate into gestational diabetes.

Your **digestive tract slows down** and gets sensitive – and this leads to a number of possible symptoms. You might also experience **cold and flu-like symptoms** and a nasal congestion because increased blood supply and oestrogen can swell up the nasal passages. Try steam, hydrating fluids and gentle exercise; elevate your head with a pillow while sleeping.

Finally, you might find yourself **spotting (or bleeding)**. Don't panic. Spotting is more common than you'd imagine; there could be multiple reasons for it (see box 'Spotting in your first trimester: What does it mean?' and box 'You've noticed heavier bleeding and you're scared: Understand the possible causes').

Most miscarriages also occur in the first trimester (see section 'Miscarriage'), so take stock of some of the signs. We'll look into a few of the rampant symptoms in detail below.

Morning sickness

There is no fixed time or pattern for these waves of nausea (dry heaving, dizziness, retching, vomiting). It can occur at any time of the day and start from early pregnancy, going even into the fourth month. For some moms, morning sickness lasts the whole nine months! It is likely to be at its highest around week eight or nine, and ease off for most women around week 12. Ask your doctor for anti-nausea medication if your symptoms are too much to handle without allopathy. Remember, excess antacids and other chemical components can restrict urine and bowel movements and add to your nausea – so take these in measured doses.

If you're too sick to eat or certain foods make you nauseous, don't worry. Small dietary additions will help: even something as simple as ginger and lemon. It's a great time to start using different foods to look after your changing body (see Chapter 8: Nutrition). An imbalance of electrolytes is normal, thanks to the vomiting and/or dehydration. Try and up your fluid intake – although it may seem like an uphill task with the nausea. Dry foods usually help; consider munching on a biscuit, dry toast, a cracker or a breadstick first thing in the morning. Attempt a banana and try and add some ginger/lemon to your diet. Sip on liquids slowly and skip greasy and sugary foods.

Some moms can suffer from a heightened form of morning sickness when the vomiting and nausea is severe or, in extreme cases, non-stop. This is a condition called **hyperemesis gravidarum,** and you will have to go to a hospital for intravenous drips and will need anti-nausea medication.

Why do I have a headache?

A lot of women find that a headache is a near-constant companion in their first trimester – even if they have never been headache-prone before. At the most basic level, it is a response to your body's elevated hormones and fluctuating blood volumes. Whether it is dull, throbbing, pulsating or one-sided, tell your doctor. It could be a tension headache induced by stress, or it may have a bearing on your blood pressure and blood sugar levels. Potentially, things like poor nutrition, dehydration, changes in vision or even certain foods can be the likely causes.

Why do I feel tired and sleepy?

Sleepiness and a feeling of tiredness are common, thanks to your body working extra to create both your baby and the little world within that is protecting it. Allow your body to rest. Your increased blood volume and progesterone is causing this. Also, disturbed sleep patterns are common if you are anxious, which makes you sleepier during the day. Moderate physical activity and good nutrition will help ease this feeling. By the end of the first 12 weeks, you are highly likely to feel energized.

Why do smells and tastes bother me?

A heightened sensitivity to smells and tastes can occur during pregnancy – if you randomly feel a gag reflex, this is probably it. Some women may have dysgeusia, when increased oestrogen and water retention alter your taste buds or bring that metallic taste to your mouth. You may feel like eating more salt, citrus and soy. Just gargle and brush more often. This feeling is harmless, and there is nothing you can do about it.

My stomach is in flux: acidity, gas, constipation, loose motions

The hormones in your body and the iron in your prenatal vitamins (see section 'What medicines do I need?') can slow down your digestion process. Acidity and gas are common. Depending on your gut, you may get constipated or get loose motions (though the former is more widespread). Now is when you reach for the fibre-rich foods and really amp up your water intake. Eat smaller portions of food more frequently and don't have tea or coffee first thing in the morning. A medley of pregnancy vitamins can wreak havoc with your intestines. So really be careful with how many pills you're popping. Try sugar-free barley water, simple nimbu pani, dahi, banana and add touches of ginger juice and lemon juice to your diet.

SPOTTING IN YOUR FIRST TRIMESTER: WHAT DOES IT MEAN?

There can be nothing scarier than to find yourself bleeding in your first trimester. IVF moms are especially prone to this. Some light bleeding is completely normal, though you must immediately consult your doctor.

1. Implantation bleeding is common within the first 12 days after conception has occurred. It most often manifests as light pink or brown spotting and mild-ish PMS symptoms (easily confused by most women to be the start of their period). Chances of implantation bleeding are more pronounced when you're pregnant with multiple babies.

2. Your cervix is a lot more sensitive with pregnancy hormones at play, which means intercourse – among other things – can cause a bit of spotting.

3. Cervical polyps (predominantly curable and largely benign) can get inflamed and cause a bleed. You need to see your ob-gyn.

4. A simple urinary tract infection (UTI) in the pelvis or bladder or a vaginal yeast infection can cause white discharge, light bleeding, a burning sensation while urinating and itchiness in the vagina or visible sores on the genitals. Your ob-gyn needs to see you to fix this.

5. There are also non-obstetric causes (ones unrelated to the pregnancy) for bleeding, like cervicitis, vaginitis, cystitis, cervical cancer, a ruptured varicose vein or polyps. Medical intervention is a must.

You've noticed heavier bleeding and you're scared: Understand the possible causes

If you notice a much heavier bleed, that is bright red, pink or brown, along with some or all of these symptoms – i.e., lower back pain, pressure in the rectum, nausea, chills, a fever, stomach cramps in sharp waves or small clots – consider it a red flag. Rush to your obstetrician/gynaecologist. It could possibly mean one of the following:

1. The start of a miscarriage, which happens most commonly within the first 12 weeks of pregnancy.

2. A 'threatened abortion', i.e., symptoms of a miscarriage without a miscarriage.

3. An ectopic pregnancy, i.e., an uncommon phenomenon when the egg embeds itself outside the womb, mainly in the fallopian tubes. An abortion is required here.

4. Gestational trophoblastic disease (GTD): Pregnancy-related rare tumours that cause unusual cell growth

in the uterus. One of the manifestations is a molar pregnancy, an abnormality in placental tissue because of a genetic error. Most such moles are surgically removable. One of the forms of GTD can be malignant.

5. Subchorionic haemorrhage or subchorionic haematoma, i.e., when the placenta detaches a little from the wall of the womb, forming a sac in the gap. It is super common, especially the small ones. A bit of bed rest usually fixes it along with doctor-prescribed medication. A large haematoma may need to be more closely monitored. Then there is retrochorionic haemorrhage that occurs behind the placenta.

6. Low implantation of the gestational sac, i.e., when the embryo implants itself in the lower section of the uterus. A low-lying placenta, preterm labour, a Caesarean delivery and, in some cases, a miscarriage are possible outcomes. Your ob-gyn will monitor you closely, repeat ultrasounds and have you rest while following nutrition precautions.

Timely medical intervention is ideal in any of these scenarios.

How will I look?

I lost three kilos in the first three months of my second pregnancy because I was severely nauseous and unable to eat. I can't say I had any such qualms during my first pregnancy! I enjoyed every minute of it – in terms of what I ate (and how much weight I gained), how I looked and felt, and how I dressed.

From the outside, your body is unlikely to change very much in shape. Most women don't gain more than two kilos in their first trimester. Some are likely to lose a couple of kilos if they're extremely nauseous and unable to eat.

The excess amounts of oestrogen, progesterone, and hCG along with increased blood volume can give your skin that flushed look often called 'pregnancy glow'. The inconvenient truth about hormones, though, is that everybody responds to them differently. While some moms will glow, these hormones can also cause an increase in oil secretion for other moms. Result? Pregnancy acne. Ugh. It is also quite likely that your pre-existing skin conditions (such as eczema, psoriasis and rosacea, to name a few) can get aggravated.

Increased body temperature can cause hot flashes or skin rash. Your nails may start growing faster and/or become brittle because of iron deficiency. Your pregnancy growth hormones will make your hair fall less; many moms love their new and improved pregnancy mane. Women have noticed altered or improved vision during their pregnancy too. The start of hyper-pigmentation (or darkening of the skin) in select places is also pretty common (see Chapter 10: Self-Care).

Don't be surprised to see excessive hair growth in areas of your body where you had little or no hair earlier. Remember, almost all of these are mere cosmetic inconveniences, and unless a symptom bothers you too much – like uncontrollable itching (which we address later in the trimester three section) – you may need minimal medical intervention.

Your emotions

During Taimur's time I was excited and felt completely energized. I travelled the world and explored things. The only thing I remember feeling anxious about, even that early on, was breastfeeding! But with Jeh, I did feel more stressed and anxious in general because I felt so ill and we were at the height of the pandemic.

Anxiety and excitement are probably your most likely companions at this point. Why would you be anxious? There are many possible reasons for pregnant women to feel stressed: the impending reality of parenthood and your changing body, financial planning, the act of birthing, breastfeeding (yes, even though it's so far away) and planning for and accommodating a baby. You may worry because you feel physically sick and temporarily incapacitated. Miscarriages may also be a real fear – over 80 per cent of miscarriages happen in the first trimester (see section 'Miscarriage').

You can have sudden bouts of crying, mood swings, meltdowns and emotional upheavals, which is nothing out of the ordinary. Your hormone levels are off the charts at the moment and have a direct bearing on how you feel.

Diet and exercise can help calm you down. Physical activity of any kind will regulate your insulin level, which means it's great for you (see Chapter 9: Fitness). Foods with good fats, antioxidants, fibre, protein and anti-inflammatory properties can help you regulate your hormones somewhat and your nerves (see Chapter 8: Nutrition). But this is a delicate time, and it will be hard to control your emotions. Don't be tough on yourself. Accept this moment, and try and surround yourself with people who love and care for you. Have positive thoughts. Remember, it will pass and that many women are, and have been, on this emotional roller coaster. You aren't alone.

Help, my anxiety is overwhelming

With Sonali Gupta, clinical psychologist

Anxiety about body weight, breastfeeding and childbirth is experienced by most pregnant women. Older moms wonder if they would be less anxious if they were younger. Young moms wonder if they are prepared enough; will they be good moms? As a to-be parent, it's normal to feel anxious and unprepared for parenthood.

As a pregnant woman, it's very normal for you to worry about the labour, the stitches and even the pain. We need to remember that anxiety as an emotion works to prepare us for what lies ahead. Begin with acknowledging your anxiety and also what is triggering it. At the same time, if anxiety is persistent and severe in intensity, it may need attention from a mental health professional.

The one thing I would advise every woman to do from the time she finds out she is pregnant is to communicate. Ask questions and don't judge yourself for the questions you have. Don't label your questions as being stupid or irrational. You would be surprised to know that when women finally speak to their partner about their fears and anxieties, they end up realizing that often they both have similar insecurities.

The idea of an ideal pregnancy brings narratives of perfection: of doing it all; of doing it right. Not just that, but a pressure to look beautiful while doing it! Try to pause and step back when you find yourself falling for the 'perfection trap'. Learn to give yourself the gift of self-compassion.

Just like a baby can soothe itself, we are innately capable of calming ourselves down and managing our own anxiety. How? Consider this checklist:

1. Engage in activities that comfort you: Painting, journalling, listening to music, taking a solitary walk or watching your favourite film again.

2. Engage in social soothing: Reach out to your partner, friend, mother or a relative whom you can trust and talk about what's bothering you. Even holding someone's hand is enough sometimes. Reaching out is a sign of strength, not weakness.

3. The simplest one? If you're pregnant with your second child, lying down next to your first child can be something which so many mothers describe as soothing and reassuring.

4. Despite trying everything, if you are still anxious and unable to sleep, consider consulting a mental health professional.

5. Be self-compassionate: You are pregnant and while what you are doing is common to a million women, that doesn't mean that it is not changing your life. It's huge and is a milestone that's special for you and your family.

Miscarriage

Some 15 to 25 per cent of discovered pregnancies result in miscarriage. The risk of a miscarriage is highest in the first trimester – 85 per cent of all miscarriages happen during this time. This number drops dramatically after women pass the 12-week mark. There is also an age-dependent risk, with women over 35 years of age being at a higher risk of miscarriage than younger women. First trimester miscarriages happen most commonly because the baby doesn't develop properly or has chromosomal defects. Other causes include an infection or a hormonal, cervical or immune system issue in the mother. Keep a careful eye on the possible signs that you may be having a miscarriage. You don't have to feel any one of these or even all of them, it could be a combination:

- Bleeding
- Severe cramping and pain in your lower abdomen (like enhanced menstrual cramps or that feeling like you want to use the toilet)
- Spasmodic pain in your lower back
- Discharge of fluid from the vagina
- Discharge of tissue/clots from the vagina
- Nausea and fatigue
- A sudden end to the pregnancy symptoms you were feeling so far (like morning sickness and so on)

What happens post the miscarriage?

Your doctor will either allow the uterine tissue to pass out naturally (or aided with medicines) or will do a procedure called dilatation and curettage (D&C). For a D&C, your doctor will widen your cervix with tools and scrape off all remaining tissue from the uterine lining in order to prevent an infection. This will ideally happen under some form of anaesthesia. Your doctor will then prescribe over-the-counter (OTC) pain relief medication to tide you over the next few days. You can commence your regular routine shortly after a miscarriage, but avoid sex and tampons. Pregnancy hormones will stay in your bloodstream for one to two months.

Miscarriages can be a time of great grief. This is the time to take help and support from friends, family or counsellors. Women often talk about not being able to show their grief publicly and the pressure it puts upon them. Don't feel guilty about seeking help if you need it. Remember too that your body will recover soon (in about a month) and that many women go on to have a healthy and safe pregnancy thereafter.

What am I allowed to do?

If you're feeling fine and energetic, and if your doctor has declared yours a safe pregnancy, you can do the things you enjoy with minimal restrictions. Exercise, travel, attend social events, have sex, go to work – life is normal. If you have a sensitive pregnancy, you will of course have to follow your doctor's advice before you make any moves. In case you have a precious pregnancy, be prepared for several restrictions; many of them may be self-imposed. It is only normal to have fears in this case. Always consult your doctor.

WHAT IS A PRECIOUS PREGNANCY?

It refers to any pregnancy that has come after a long wait, after medical treatment or with a significant risk factor like the age and health of the mother; foetal complications; etc. Why is a precious pregnancy considered delicate? One, complications are involved. Two, the parents-to-be are stressed. Three, there is a much larger component of medical intervention involved through the pregnancy. Four, friends, family and doctors feel the need to be overprotective and overcautious about this pregnancy. Physically, emotionally, socially and financially, a lot of factors come into play in such a pregnancy.

Sex

Are you feeling nervous about having sex? Worried that you might harm your baby or cause a miscarriage? Don't worry, it is completely safe to have sex during your first trimester. If you are on pelvic rest for any reason, it is best to seek your doctor's advice. If you had sex and find you're spotting or bleeding, don't panic. Your cervix is remodelling itself during this stage of your pregnancy and is tender. Wear a sanitary napkin and speak to your doctor.

The hormones ruling your body will also affect your sex drive – while some moms talk about an increased libido, others often have no sex drive whatsoever. Find different ways to feel pleasure then. More than anything, say no to your partner if you really don't feel like it.

A good orgasm will quite likely make you feel better. Keep it gentle and find positions that don't terrify you. Issues like changes in your pelvic floor muscles, hormone fluxes, a feeling of tightness, extra lubrication, sensitive genitalia and more are common to women across varying ages, making intercourse a little easier or more strained. Oral sex is also safe, though a very commonly understood thumb rule is: do not blow air directly into the vagina. This is a risk factor for an air embolism.

Exercise

Yes! Physical activity is very beneficial for you during pregnancy and for your growing foetus. Walk and swim and climb those flights of stairs. It is great to regulate your blood flow, balance your insulin level and generally feel more energized and fit. If you have a healthy pregnancy, your doctor won't stop you from doing most exercises except for the ones where you might be in danger of falling – say, cycling out on the street. Some experts recommend cycling (in the gym) or swimming – over walking – because both are non-weight-bearing exercises.

However, as anyone will tell you, now is definitely not the time to start anything new. The main rule of thumb for exercising while pregnant is to continue to do things that you already know. If you haven't exercised and want to start, start by walking and then discuss with your doctor. If you've always been active at a gym, use the gym machines you are already accustomed to, with free weights and treadmills.

For yoga or Pilates, work with a certified prenatal trainer or inform your instructor that you're pregnant so your workouts can be tweaked accordingly. Are you working out or doing yoga with ready online videos? Switch to pregnancy videos.

Eating

On the whole, eat how you always ate. Think healthy and fresh; stick to smaller portions if you need to. You may be pressured by family members to suddenly start eating more, but follow the signs your body gives you. You'll be told that 'you're eating for two now', but you're not.

There may be too much nausea for you to be able to eat. Go easy. What you could begin to avoid is alcohol, less than even two drinks a week is recommended in pregnancy (see box 'Alcohol consumption'). And go easy on caffeine (200 mg per day is the global recommendation; see Chapter 8: Nutrition). If you're into aerated soft drinks, now would be a really good time to stop as the sugar and caffeine content is high. Stop cigarettes and packaged foods (packed wafers, popcorn, bottled sauces, ready-to-eat items and so on), so that you can start taking careful stock of your salt and sugar intake from direct and indirect sources. This has a bearing on things that could bother you later – like pregnancy-induced hypertension, pre-eclampsia, gestational diabetes, joint pain or swollen limbs.

Pregnant women are known to be sensitive to food-borne illnesses and gastroenteritis or even a simple runny tummy.

Unpasteurized milk is basically raw and untreated milk from any animal. It can contain harmful bacteria like listeria, salmonella and E. Coli. Before consuming any dairy-based products, check if the milk it contains is pasteurized or not. Most of us today do not bring unpasteurized milk home.

As per global standards, avoid mould-ripened soft cheese (brie, camembert, chevre, ricotta, cottage, Danish blue, gorgonzola) because these contain bacteria (listeria) which could be harmful. If you have that cheese craving, stick to hard ones (cheddar, parmesan) or soft pasteurized ones (paneer, mozzarella). Cheese and dairy products derived from pasteurized milk – like homemade paneer, dahi, chaas – are safe.

Remember one golden rule in pregnancy eating, given your sensitized digestive tract. Any food that has travelled very far to get on to your plate – especially highly perishable items like imported cheese, yogurt, butter and ice cream – are avoidable. These items need to be transferred and stored at a reliable temperature until the time they come to your home. And that doesn't always happen. In the process, they can breed bacteria like listeria and other pathogens that can upset your stomach.

You could avoid raw foods (raw milk, uncooked egg, raw seafood, cold-cut meats, salad, juices). Some of them, like salad and juice, hamper your delicate digestive tract, while others can be hazardous owing to bacteria. Ensure your food is well cooked because your pregnancy hormones and multivitamins have already sensitized your gut.

Up to three weekly servings of cooked, low-mercury seafood is good. Nearly all types of seafood has small amounts of mercury, but some large, predatory fish like shark, swordfish, king mackerel or tuna have it in higher quantities. If mercury levels accumulate in your body, it can harm your baby and its delicate and developing nervous system. It is unlikely that this should be a problem for most of you, though – one, you will need to have a large amount of these fish to get affected; two, these are not foods we typically consume. However, tuna is a common fish, so if you are a regular tuna fish eater, be very mindful of how much you eat.

People will have a list of suggestions on fruits and vegetables that must be avoided during pregnancy, but you can't go wrong if you consume in moderation and think homemade, well-cooked, simple, seasonal, local (see Chapter 8: Nutrition).

ALCOHOL CONSUMPTION

While it may be ideal to avoid alcohol during pregnancy, your doctor may allow you to consume one to two units of alcohol in a week. This is a global standard. Now, what do these units mean?

- 1 x standard glass of wine (175 ml) = 2.1 units
- 1 x 25 ml shot of spirits = 1 unit
- 1 can of beer = 2 units

Can I travel?

If your ob-gyn is satisfied that you have a healthy pregnancy under way (and if you are adequately energetic), he/she is likely to clear you for travel. There is an equally good chance that your ob-gyn and sonologist may be a little conservative in their views on travel at any point of time in your pregnancy. It's absolutely fine. You have to assess this situation for yourself. Why the hesitation? Simply because if anything were to go wrong – like, say, you developed a sudden bleed – while you're on the move, on the road or in a foreign country, you would be away from your doctor and support system.

Usually your doctor will have you do an ultrasound before you leave town and again soon after you come back. There are certain parameters your sonologist may assess every time you choose to travel across all three trimesters – your cervical length, your placenta placement and the funnelling of your cervix (here, the doctor puts gentle pressure on the fundus of the uterus to see if the cervix opens up, i.e., funnels). If these parameters aren't satisfactory, your doctor may warn you against travelling. A few conditions where your doctor may advise that travel is best avoided is in case of bleeding, twin pregnancy, a history of preterm delivery/miscarriage and a precious pregnancy.

If you avoid junk food, hydrate well and walk around the airplane cabin every so often, a long flight is safe. Take breaks every three hours on a road journey where you can walk around for a few minutes and then resume your car ride. Your doctor may put you on a couple of additional medicine supplements (possibly progesterone, if needed) to tide you through your trip. Stick to safe destinations and always keep your prescribed medication (and SOS medicine for gas, nausea and a reliable paracetamol) in your handbag. Take your pregnancy vitamins diligently. In case you have always wondered, body scanners at security checkpoints are safe for pregnant women to go through. The level of radiation you are exposed to is very low. What you could do is inform the lady who scans passengers with a handheld scanning wand that you're pregnant. She may choose to avoid using it or be extra gentle around your abdomen.

(With inputs from Dr Mitossh Ruparel)

What can't I do?

Since the first trimester is when the baby is actually forming – cells, tissues, organs, bones, skin, heart and all – we tend to 'be careful'. It's quite likely your family will ask you to take it easy, rest, stay home or eat more. But there is nothing you cannot do.

There are some unhealthy habits that you should give up at this point. Smoking is a significant no-no. Most women choose to completely abstain or go super easy on caffeine and alcohol. Avoid very hot showers, sauna rooms or hot tub soaks in trimester one as it affects your body temperature and therefore your blood pressure, which could reduce blood flow to the baby. You also shouldn't be having massages during this trimester. Hair colour and special hair treatments are generally avoided in the first 12 weeks. Culturally, we are also superstitious about this time and refrain from making announcements.

There are two global cautions for pregnancy! First, changing kitty litter boxes. If you have a cat, remember that it can transmit a disease called toxoplasmosis, which can create problems for babies. You will need to make a decision on your cat with your doctor's advice. Second, avoid X-rays completely. If, for any reason, you absolutely have to get one, you will need to exercise complete precaution and follow your doctor's directives.

What happens at the doctor's?

It is critical to be comfortable with your doctor. Even through my second pregnancy, which was during the height of the pandemic, my doctor maintained that while he wanted me to be safe, he did not want to stop me from anything.

Your doctor will probably see you once a month in your first trimester. Here is a quick look at the schedule most doctors will largely follow with pregnant women – give or take a few extra appointments:

1. Once a month till 28 weeks
2. Once in two weeks from 28 weeks till 36 weeks
3. Once a week after 36 weeks till your delivery

When you choose a doctor, pick someone you feel truly comfortable with and whose outlook matches yours. You should be able to ask your doctor anything – even if you think it is a foolish question. There are many old-fashioned doctors who do not discuss too many details with their patients. Don't be embarrassed to look for someone else if you feel you need to. Above all, don't fear your doctor. Feel free to question him/her about anything that's happening to you. Why are you being put on bed rest? Can you still play tennis? Should you eat all the food your mother or mother-in-law is making you eat? Are all sex positions safe? Do you really need progesterone supplements?

In your early visits you can expect the most preliminary examination: height, weight, blood pressure, a quick physical abdominal check and your medical history. At this point, it is ideal to prepare your health history, including records of your past surgeries/illnesses, recent blood work, up-to-date immunization records, a list of your current medication and a record of your last period. Your doctor will ask you for this information.

In many cases, the doctor will do an endo-vaginal ultrasound or pelvic ultrasound as the baby might be too small for an abdominal ultrasound (see section 'A breakdown of your first trimester ultrasounds'). This helps your doctor gauge the health of your reproductive organs, see your pelvis shape, and check if your pregnancy is normal or ectopic. There is a possibility that you will be prescribed your first abdominal scan at week seven or eight, with no preceding endo-vaginal scan.

Most ob-gyns will refer you to a sonologist for your ultrasounds. Your sonologist is an equally important part of your pregnancy process. He/She will be examining you and your baby with the utmost care and precision. Your sonologist's readings are a key part of your ob-gyn's assessment and protocol for you.

For IVF moms, your IVF doctor will perform your early ultrasounds. The gestational age of your pregnancy and your due date will be given to you post the first abdominal ultrasound. For extra caution, your doctor may suggest a foetal Doppler ultrasound to detect the movement of blood in the baby's vessels. A more commonly conducted Doppler in the early stages of pregnancy, till trimester two, is to study the uterine arteries of the mother and make sure they're doing their work (see section 'A breakdown of your first trimester ultrasounds') – rather than a foetal Doppler.

What tests will I need to take?

Be prepared for a list of blood tests and a urine test to check everything from your blood group and Rh status and blood sugar to infection levels, WBC, proteins, bacteria, STDs and anaemia. Here is a comprehensive blood test list prescribed at your **first** prenatal doctor visit:

- Blood group and Rh factor
- Beta hCG – for the levels of human chorionic gonadotropin
- Serum progesterone
- FT3, FT4, TSH – for thyroid
- HCV – Hepatitis C antibody testing
- CBC – for infections
- VDRL – for venereal diseases, like syphilis
- Random blood sugar, Hb1ac – for your blood sugar levels
- HBsAG – for Hepatitis B
- HIV
- Serum iron, serum ferritin – for a complete iron profile
- Haemoglobin electrophoresis – to measure different types of haemoglobin in your bloodstream
- TORCH 10 – a profile of tests to detect presence of or immunity to viruses like herpes, toxoplasma, cytomegalovirus, rubella and other pathogens
- If you have had a planned pregnancy, you probably might already have done preconception carrier screening to check if you're a carrier for a single-gene/genetic disease like cystic fibrosis, sickle cell anaemia, thalassemia, etc. If not, your doctor will advise you on what needs to be done, often based on anomalies detected in some of the other tests. This is not a compulsory test

All the test lists presented across trimesters one, two and three are comprehensive long-lists of all possible tests and their stipulated time frames. If you have a healthy and safe pregnancy, your ob-gyn is quite likely to have you skip some of these tests

and only do what he/she deems necessary for your particular case. If you have questions around these, ask your doctor.

Apart from the blood tests:
- Urine test – can be indicative of infection, proteins, pre-eclampsia and gestational diabetes
- Blood pressure – must be regularly checked to monitor the risk of pre-eclampsia (dangerously high blood pressure) and pregnancy-induced hypertension

A breakdown of your first trimester ultrasounds

Saif and I were always excited about going together for my scans. Before you wonder, I can tell you we were never bothered about finding out the sex of either of our babies.

There are typically two ways in which an ultrasound examination (also called a sonography) is carried out during your first trimester: endo-vaginal and abdominal. In the early stages of your pregnancy, an endo-vaginal ultrasound is done. A fresh condom is unwrapped and placed on a wand-shaped transducer with lubrication. This is gently inserted into your vagina. It may feel uncomfortable but it will not hurt. This probe emits sound waves to obtain high-resolution images. All your subsequent ultrasounds will then be abdominal ultrasounds, where a special gel will be rubbed on your bare abdomen and a small probe-like transducer will be placed on top of the gel to use high-frequency sound waves to capture live images from inside your body.

One of the foremost worries amongst most new moms is about whether there is any radiation involved in an ultrasound and if it would cause the baby any harm. The answer is, no. Ultrasound waves are not harmful to the baby. Note: Dress in a two-piece outfit for your ultrasound as far as possible so your doctor can access your abdomen with minimal fuss. It will be easier for you!

• The first ultrasound scan is done at around six to seven weeks after you've missed your period. Your doctor will do an endo-vaginal ultrasound to determine if you're pregnant or not. Visualisation of the gestational sac inside the uterus confirms the pregnancy. At around five weeks, the gestational sac is the first structure to appear, followed by the yolk sac and the embryo at six weeks. On visualization of heart activity in the embryo, your doctor declares your pregnancy as viable and healthy. Your sonologist will check for the position of the sac and also the number of sacs to determine if you have more than one baby. The doctor will also determine the exact duration of your pregnancy and give you your expected due date.

• The second primary ultrasound is an abdominal ultrasound. This is called the nuchal translucency (NT) scan and it is done between 11 and 13 weeks. It is specifically done when the length of the foetus is between 45 and 84 mm. NT is an important scan for screening chromosomal abnormalities. It basically measures the thickness of the fluid build-up at the back of the baby's neck. If this area is thicker than normal, it can be an early sign of Down syndrome, trisomy 18 or heart problems.

The NT is done along with the important '**double marker**'/'**dual plus**' blood test (also referred to as maternal serum screening). This test reveals if there is an increased risk of chromosomal anomalies in the foetus by screening your levels of beta-hCG, estriol and pregnancy-associated plasma protein A (PAPP-A). Based on these readings, your ob-gyn and sonologist will advise you further.

While an ultrasound combined with the dual marker blood test is a lot more common, you can choose to opt for NIPS or NIPT – i.e., non-invasive prenatal screening/testing. This blood test is ideally done at 10 weeks of pregnancy. It is an expensive but an effective, accurate and safe method for detecting chromosomal abnormalities in the unborn baby. In case your dual marker test and ultrasound reflect questionable results, your doctor may suggest NIPT (see box 'Confused on blood tests and NIPT? Let's understand what is happening here').

CONFUSED ON BLOOD TESTS AND NIPT? LET'S UNDERSTAND WHAT IS HAPPENING HERE

You will have a blood biomarker test each in trimester one ('dual plus' at 11–13 weeks) and trimester two ('quadruple marker' at 16–22 weeks), largely combined with an ultrasound both times. Both these tests are meant to assess the risk of chromosomal anomalies in the foetus. However, if you are an older mom or have a precious pregnancy – or even if you'd just like to err on the side of caution at an early stage – you can opt for NIPS or NIPT, i.e., a non-invasive prenatal screening test.

NIPT basically isolates the cell-free DNA (cfDNA) in the mother's blood and analyses it for chromosomal anomalies. Globally, NIPT has often shown near-accurate sensitivity. It is ideal to opt for NIPT at about 10 weeks of pregnancy. The advantage of diagnosing this early is: (a) it assesses your baby's genetic health, (b) it opens up several options for further testing, (c) it gives you time to assess the viability of your pregnancy, (d) it can avoid invasive procedures like amniocentesis and chorionic villus sampling later on in pregnancy. NIPT is not a very commonly prescribed test as it is expensive. Ask your doctor about laboratories that conduct NIPT in India.

3D and 4D Ultrasounds: What do they really mean?

3D is when multiple 2D images of your baby are pieced together to make a 3D image for you. And when you can also see the 3D images of your baby moving (i.e., in real time), like in a video, it is 4D. Most doctors will prescribe one such scan in your 40 weeks; usually **between 24 and 28 weeks** (sometimes doctors opt for 3D/4D scans to detect foetal anomalies, spinal cord issues, and so on). There is no harm to your baby in terms of sound waves – while the technology and the probe may differ, the sound waves in 2D, 3D and 4D are the same. The cost, however, is vastly different.

Kareena was an amazing patient. Of course I loved her movies, but meeting her in person made me even more fond of her. She was normal, down-to-earth and she walked in and out of my clinic like any other patient. She took most appointments herself; she'd message me first before calling and would always seek an appointment from me at a time convenient to both of us. Saif accompanied her during Taimur's time for two or three scans. But she also often came alone.

She was very particular and followed her ultrasound schedule to the T. She would work her important scans around her trips and shoots. I have an extra monitor on the ceiling in my clinic so my patient can see the scans clearly. And I remember she would be completely absorbed by my commentary and in watching the baby on the screen above her. I tend to explain everything to my patients – the anatomical structures and the physiology of the baby; how the baby sips amniotic fluid and passes urine. There was this gleam in her eye the whole time and a smile on her face. She was just so happy to know that the baby was all right – that's all she wanted to hear. I remember her last ultrasound during Taimur's time. She came with Saif and they asked if they could take a selfie with me – just to commemorate their last scan before their baby arrived. Saif and she were just so content with each other, and so thrilled about their babies. – DR MITOSSH RUPAREL, sonologist

What medicines do I need?

I put myself on folic acid the minute I found out I was pregnant until I finished my first trimester during Taimur's and Jeh's pregnancies. I supplemented my vitamin intake with this amazing multivitamin called PregnaCare with an extra 1000 mg dose of calcium. Folic acid, calcium and PregnaCare were my companions through both my pregnancies. I had to use anti-nausea medication in my second pregnancy, but I strictly stuck to my doctor's prescriptions.

There are no medicines required through trimester one. However you will have to most likely take a few supplements. A folic acid supplement is important in the first trimester because it can assist in avoiding significant neural tube defects in the foetus. Your doctor may ask you to stop folic acid post your 12- to 14-week mark.

Apart from folic acid, your doctor may put you on additional vitamin supplements. A pregnancy multivitamin contains a mix of vitamins B1, B2, B3, B6, B12, C, D, E, K, folic acid, iodine, magnesium, iron, copper, zinc and selenium – depending on the brand. If you have already been consuming some of these multivitamins, you can stick to the same. A pregnancy multivitamin is a rebranded, repackaged one-stop shop, which makes it attractive for the user.

A booster dose of calcium, iron and vitamin D is often recommended by doctors. In fact, a lot of doctors ask their pregnant patients to continue their calcium supplements till six months post delivery. If your progesterone levels seem low (or your doctor foresees any risk to your pregnancy), a progesterone supplement might be prescribed to you. These come in the form of injections, oral pills or a vaginal suppository and sometimes might make you feel tired. Many IVF moms will be put on a progesterone regimen in the first trimester. Medication to modulate your blood sugar levels (i.e., metformin) is also a possibility, if your blood work indicates an unhappy level of blood sugar.

If you are already on medication, your doctor may ask you to stop or switch medicines at this time. Most women do not even pop a paracetamol without consulting their doctor first, and that is probably the most commonly used medication in pregnancy for a pain, fever or cold. Many antibiotics are safe, but there are also exceptions to this list. Bear in mind your medicine allergies. Simple OTC drugs are considered safe, but – for instance – every available antacid may not be good for you. It depends on the chemical components of each. It would be best to consult your ob-gyn before you pop any pill. The chemical component or steroid component in many OTC drugs may be unsafe for pregnancy too. Some medicines can be teratogenic, which means it can cause defects in the baby. Do not self-medicate during pregnancy.

It is a good time to start a pregnancy file where you can keep track of your supplements and/or required vaccinations as the doctor prescribes. Make notes of your medicines, when and how to consume your vitamins, your nausea patterns, cravings and also just your moods and thoughts.

How do I optimize the absorption of all my vitamins?

With Dr Rita Shah, Lamaze consultant and director of Nine Months, a fitness and guidance programme for expectant mothers

A lot of women think they will 'forget' their vitamins and therefore choose to pop all of them at one go every day. But these medicines don't get absorbed into your body very well if you consume all of them together. As a rule of thumb, for instance, never combine iron and calcium supplements. Instead, you can safely take your folic acid tablet with iron. Calcium works just fine as a stand-alone tablet. It is best absorbed on a full gut, which is why most moms prefer to have it after a good dinner. There are a select few, however, who cannot tolerate calcium at night; consult your doctor in that case and consider taking it on an empty stomach in the morning. Your doctor may also recommend a good time of day to take the calcium supplement.

Iron is a difficult element to be taken in by the body. Some get loose motions; some get constipated. In case you cannot tolerate a specific supplement, let your doctor change the medicine or the formulation you're consuming. Iron levels tend to drop as your pregnancy progresses. Keep up with your supplements to avoid iron injections or intravenous iron drips (both these options are painful). Iron can be consumed at any time of the day and it is best had with a glass of citrus juice. So squeeze out a few drops of lemon juice into a glass of water to swallow your iron pill. Many moms choose to have a tablet of vitamin C with their iron tablet.

Remember when it comes to consuming vitamins and supplements, there are always small exceptions to the norm. It is not okay to suffer through several bouts of loose motions a day because you're consuming all these pills. It will do you more harm than good.

Complications of trimester one

You could have severe leg pain or severe headaches, low implantation of the gestational sac or a miscarriage. Then there is bleeding/spotting, burning during urination, vaginal discharge or itching and excessive nausea. There can also be a flare-up of pre-existing skin conditions or chronic diseases and stress. As we've discussed earlier in this chapter, these are some of the possible complications of trimester one. But let's look in detail at a rare condition called thrombosis, which may commence with an appearance of a clot during trimester one.

Thrombosis/Embolism

Yes, it can happen. No, it doesn't happen to everyone. In fact, it is a rather uncommon occurrence. But, between a pregnant and non-pregnant woman, a pregnant woman is about five times likelier to develop a clot. It means she is 'hypercoagulable'. Studies show a clot can form during the first trimester of pregnancy, during childbirth, or up to about six weeks post delivery.

Thrombosis is a blood clot that forms in a vein. It is called venous thrombosis. When it forms in a vein that is deep below your skin's surface, it is called DVT (or deep vein thrombosis). DVT is the most common pregnancy clot. Signs of DVT? Leg or calf pain, swelling, redness; large-looking veins on legs; warmth in clot areas; a pain that increases if you walk. Clots can travel through your body – to your lung or brain. And this is what makes them a significant risk, even post delivery.

What makes you more susceptible to clots currently and through your pregnancy later? If you are an older mom, have been overweight, a smoker, on bed rest, on a long flight, have a family history of blood clots, have thrombophilia (i.e., your blood is more likely to clot), and haven't been physically active during pregnancy.

Symptoms are breathlessness; blood in cough; chest pain; breathing difficulty; blue skin; signs of a stroke; mental confusion; low blood pressure; significant muscle or joint pain. It is best to seek medical help immediately.

What can a first trimester SOS visit to your ob-gyn entail?

1. A proper physical examination and breakdown of your symptoms
2. An ultrasound (endo-vaginal scan in the very early part of your pregnancy and an abdominal scan later)
3. A blood test or urine test to check for hCG levels, infection and other anomaly markers
4. A Doppler ultrasound to detect the movement of blood in vessels and hence measure blood flow in the placenta, umbilical cord and the body of the foetus (In the earlier stages of your pregnancy your sonologist will not opt for a foetal Doppler unless it is required to check on your baby. The Doppler machine uses a higher frequency of sound waves than the ultrasound machine.)

Preparations for trimester one

Is there a shopping list?

Take a deep breath. There are no shopping lists. Your baby and you don't need anything at the moment. Do you need to reach for those maternity pants? No. Most women's bodies change minimally in trimester one.

Do I need to prepare for my pregnancy at home?

Not immediately, as your life and requirements will not change right away. But it's a good time to start the thread of conversation with your partner and with your family on how you plan to incorporate this baby into your life – in terms of physical space, finances; how you wish to birth and where; who your obstetrician/gynaecologist will be; and how you would like your family to be involved in your pregnancy and childbirth.

When do I announce my pregnancy?

Saif and I waited till we inched into my second trimester to announce the pregnancy, both times. Everyone just felt I was looking bigger than normal. We didn't make any grand announcements on social media, but when he was questioned about it by journalists or friends, he said we were expecting a baby. It was all very casual. But Saif is like that, understated and private.

Friends and family: Most Indian families don't announce their pregnancies till the first trimester has safely passed (and the anomaly screening has been done). This is mainly because apart from the fact that a baby bump is barely visible anyway, miscarriage risks drop sharply post the first 12 weeks of pregnancy. People tend to be superstitious about the first trimester as a critical component of the baby's development happens during this phase. Depending on how you're doing – in terms of your blood pressure, any spotting or bleeding, dizzy spells and so on – your doctor will prescribe rest or let you roam free. Figure out a strong backup excuse for any of the social events you may be missing! Either way, in India, culturally, ultimate care is taken during the first three months of pregnancy.

At work: When it comes to your workplace, you can decide when you want to share your news. Unless you're particularly sick and need time off, there is no obligation to announce your pregnancy or due date until your first trimester has passed. But it is important to take stock of how the next year is looking for you professionally; based on the hierarchy and your role in the organization and, more importantly, your profession. You need to see what works best. For instance, if you were being considered for a new role in the organization, you're a performer (theatre, film), you had travel commitments, a career transition or your work is sensitive, you may need to speak to someone about your pregnancy this early on.

REGISTERING FOR YOUR DELIVERY

Depending on your doctor, you will be delivering your baby at a hospital or at a nursing home. Based on the norms that the hospital/nursing home follows, you will be required to register in advance for the birth of your baby. Your doctor will guide you in the registration process. At what stage of your pregnancy you register depends on the hospital/nursing home's policy. At most private hospitals in Indian cities, you pay a deposit at the end of trimester one and then pay room charges at 28 weeks. Some places accept registrations during the seventh month of pregnancy.

End of trimester one: Quick look

Baby: Your baby is three inches long, 28–29 grams in weight and almost looks like a tiny formed human. This trimester is critical to the baby's growth.

Mom: You look the same on the outside – most women don't gain more than two kilos in the first trimester. But your body is churning non-stop within, and many of you may feel exhausted and nauseous through this time. The good news is that the hard bit is mostly over, and you are about to step into the easiest and most enjoyable part of your pregnancy.

2

YOUR SECOND TRIMESTER

I worked the most during my second trimesters during both my pregnancies. And I travelled the most. With Taimur, I went to Rome, Florence and Pataudi, and with Jeh, I did Dharamshala and Palampur. In Jeh's time, despite the pandemic, I shot a film and did a radio show. In fact, I commuted from Delhi to Pataudi every day while shooting for my film Laal Singh Chaddha *– just so that I could be at home with Saif and Taimur. I wrapped up almost all my professional commitments by the end of trimester two. I don't think I had time to think or prepare for my kids until I reached trimester three because I kept myself so busy!*

Congratulations again – you've made it through the first stretch of your pregnancy and are now in what most women find is their mellow zone! For most of you, those first trimester symptoms – like fatigue, nausea, headaches, spotting and tender breasts – have eased. It's a great relief. You are quite likely to feel energetic and active.

Your second trimester is the fourth, fifth and sixth months of your pregnancy, from week 14 till week 28. This is when your baby's organs are fully formed and continually developing, and the little one is a miniature version of what she'll be when she comes out into the world. Your baby bump will begin to grow, and by the end of this trimester most of you will be showing. You will see changes in your weight as well. And there are some fun developments too – your baby will start to move, and you may feel her butterfly flutters, somewhere mid-trimester.

The second trimester doesn't have the anxieties or the symptoms of trimester one. Your baby is stable and secure in your womb now, but she is also still too little to bring you those feelings of discomfort that will occur in the later stages of your pregnancy.

On the flip side, you may feel one or more of the following: the occasional sharp stomach pain on the sides, leaky breasts, stuffy nose, itchy abdomen and darkening of skin in places. Plus, be prepared for heartburn, joint aches and clumsiness (butterfingers, anyone?)! You're wondering, 'But I thought this would be easy!' Don't worry, despite these symptoms, most moms-to-be find these three months the easiest and most relaxing. Many of you may not experience most of these symptoms. And none of them are as exhausting as the nausea and fatigue that hit most women in trimester one.

Many of you will feel a renewed sense of positivity about your pregnancy, especially now that the risk of miscarriage has reduced. This is also the time when most of you will announce the pregnancy to friends, family and colleagues, and it can be a relief to finally share this big news with everyone. Based on the cultural beliefs of your family, be prepared for black threads, amulets or bands to be tied to your wrist, ankle or around your neck during this phase.

Surprisingly, some women get more worried because there

may be a sudden disappearance of those first trimester symptoms. Am I still pregnant, you might wonder? How come it's all disappeared? Remember, many women feel as you do and there is usually nothing to worry about. But if those worries don't go away, talk to your ob-gyn, sonologist and family doctor.

Vaccines, ultrasounds and critical blood tests (like the quadruple marker and the glucose test) are an important element of trimester two. Focus on looking after yourself this trimester: eat well, stay mobile, have your vitamins, plan for the future and enjoy your growing baby. The reality of your pregnancy will also hit you and your partner at this stage. You can actually just use this time to start talking about the new addition to your family and ease into the realities of what life is going to be like.

Your second trimester is also an important milestone in terms of preterm births. If your baby is born prematurely at 28 weeks and thereafter, she will have a very high chance of survival. The American Association of Pediatricians says a baby born at 28 weeks will have over 90 per cent chance of making it. Advances in medicine mean even premature babies born at 26 weeks have a strong chance of making it. While premature births will most likely be extremely upsetting and overwhelming for parents, feel reassured to know that by 28 weeks your baby is developed enough to be able to survive outside of your uterus – as long as she has access to 24x7 quality medical care (see box 'Premature babies').

A look at the second trimester for an IVF mom

An IVF pregnancy is officially considered to be no different from a normal pregnancy beyond the first few weeks post conception. It is normal to be a little more anxious if you're an IVF mom, but you are also over the delicate period and can begin to relax now. You can expect one additional routine ultrasound per trimester if you're an IVF mom; and likely a couple of extra ultrasounds if you are carrying multiple babies so that each baby can be examined. The rest of your medical protocol remains unchanged. If you have a precious pregnancy, a high-risk pregnancy, you're an older mom or are carrying multiple babies, you are much more likely to be placed under stricter cautions.

BUMP CHECK: ARE YOU HAVING A BOY OR A GIRL? PREDICTIONS, ANYONE?

It is quite likely that the minute your bump starts growing, especially as you move into your third trimester, various aunts, uncles, neighbours, relatives and grandmas will start making predictions on the gender of your baby. If your bump is high you're having a girl. If it's lower, then it's a boy. Gender predictions will also commence with observations on your skin, hair, nails, breast size (Yes! If your breasts don't get too big, you're having a boy), morning sickness, food cravings and mood swings! Take it with a pinch of salt. There is no proper scientific evidence that backs this up.

PREMATURE BABIES

A baby born any time before 37 weeks of gestation is called a premature baby or a preterm birth. The World Health Organization (WHO) says there are 15 million babies born prematurely around the world, and that this number is growing. Most premature birth babies have health complications. Many of these are short term and resolve in due course of time. (Developmentally, preterm babies catch up with full-term babies by the age of two years.) Very premature babies might have long-lasting health concerns. While there is a good chance for babies born at about 26 weeks – and, indeed, even earlier – to survive, babies born at 28 weeks and after not only have excellent chances of surviving but may grow up to have no long-lasting adverse health conditions. The most important thing to remember is that the science around this is continually developing and there will be new advances every year.

Moreover, doctors don't always know why a baby is born premature, and thus you can't usually prevent it from happening. Any number of reasons may lead to a premature birth: like an infection in the mom's body, cervical inconsistency, placenta/uterus problems, multiple babies, gestational diabetes or pre-eclampsia and so on. More recently, air pollution has been linked to premature births. For moms with a prior history of premature birth, there is a high chance of recurrence. You will need to restrict physical activity and will need injections/medicines to prevent preterm labour. Personal hygiene (preventing vaginal and urinary infections) is actually very important. See your doctor if you notice any untoward symptoms.

All premature babies require complicated medical care and an extended stay in the neonatal intensive care unit (NICU). Micropreemies (those who are born before 26 weeks) will be very thin, tiny and extremely delicate. All their in vitro milestones are achieved in the NICU, under 24x7 supervision, extensive medical care, many treatments (often invasive) and breathing/cardiac support.

Before a premature baby is discharged from the hospital and sent home with you, she has to be able to eat, breathe and stay warm without any external help. Twins born prematurely will have more complications than a singleton.

What's happening to your body in the second trimester?

I gained the maximum weight during trimester two in both my pregnancies and – let's be honest – it's also when I pigged out the most. There's no two ways about it. But I managed to find the strength to stay active – I could work and travel. And do it all!

This is the trimester where your baby really grows, your uterus expands (pushing against its surroundings to make space for itself) and your bump begins to show.

You should be **gaining 0.2 to 0.5 kg a week** in your second trimester. For mums pregnant with twins, **an approximate 0.75 kg weight gain per week is considered normal**. On an average, trimester two is when you spike on the weighing scale. A lot of women find their weight gain starts to even out again during trimester three. But everyone has a different pregnancy, and each body reacts differently to hormonal changes.

For many, your breasts may start becoming larger. It is the combination of hormonal changes with increased blood flow to your breast tissue and glands. Fat also builds up in the breast and milk glands start getting enlarged, in anticipation of lactation. Your breasts may also feel heavier and more sensitive to the touch. Well-supporting bras and hot water fomentation will help. If you see any stains on your bra, don't fret! It is colostrum, i.e., a thick yellowish substance that will leak from your breasts. It's the earliest milk produced by the mammary glands and is the first milk that your baby will have when you nurse her. While it seems like it is still too early for this, some women begin to first leak colostrum in trimester two.

This is also the time when your umbilical cord continues to thicken. It is, after all, carrying all the nourishment to your baby. Apart from this, a bunch of your normal parameters will **increase** gradually. Here is what that means: (a) your heart rate may be up 15 per cent to 20 per cent, (b) your oxygen consumption also increases 20 per cent to 40 per cent during the course of your pregnancy, to keep up with your body's metabolism and your growing baby's needs, (c) your total blood volume increases 30 per cent to 50 per cent during pregnancy, most of which happens in trimester two, (d) the metabolic rate of your body increases significantly from 15 weeks till you reach trimester three. You'll likely be feeling a lot warmer and also sweating more than the person next to you as a result. Many moms (and there is no exaggeration here) choose to sleep buck naked through the night – that is how annoyingly hot your body may feel!

Early on into this trimester, around **week 14**, your uterus, which was formerly the size of an orange located deep in your pelvis, starts ballooning outwards, leading to a lot of symptoms.

Have you rolled over in your sleep and woken up suddenly because of a sharp tugging pain in your abdomen? Random pains on the sides of your stomach are fairly common from **week 15**, since your womb is stretching. It is quite likely round ligament pain, which shows up around trimester two (see section 'How will I feel: Symptoms of trimester two').

As you go into **week 16**, your doctor will measure your blood pressure at every visit to keep a close eye on signals of rising blood pressure as it could have implications (like pre-eclampsia and pregnancy-induced hypertension) on the rest of your pregnancy. The normal range is between 110/70 and 120/80. If you're 140/90 or higher on two or more occasions, you will likely be categorized in the high blood pressure range.

By **week 17**, your placenta will grow as your baby grows and will be giving your baby all the nutrition she needs from your body. (It is interesting to note that your placenta will weigh in at about 0.45 kg by the time you reach the end of term.) **Don't be surprised, however, if your waist stops being a waist.** Things begin to look really real by now! You could also be amp-ed up on that pregnancy glow (for many of you, it's simply a flush because your body is getting hot).

From **week 18**, you could **start taking a weekly photo to track your growing belly. It's a fun way to remember the pregnancy and how your body is changing**. Remember, some women don't show until well into their fifth month too; so don't get stressed if you feel your bump is much smaller than that of some of the other to-be-moms (see box 'Is my baby growing?').

After **week 19**, your uterus is continuing to grow at the rate of around a centimetre per week.* Soon the top of your uterus

---

* It is interesting to see how the uterus measurements that your doctor takes are relevant. At your ultrasound, the doctor will measure the length between your pubic bone and the top of the uterus – which is called the 'fundus'. On your ultrasound report, you will see it noted as will be sitting roughly where your belly button is. The placenta inside your uterus also moves up and away from your cervix as your uterus grows. This is one of the things your doctor will be monitoring during your ultrasounds. Don't worry, however, if you have a low-lying placenta (called placenta previa) at this stage. Right now, it does not have any implications on a future preterm birth or a Caesarean delivery. But your doctor will advise you to curtail your activity to avoid unnecessary bleeding. Around **week 20**, many mums feel their baby's movements for the first time. These little flutters of movement are called 'quickening' (see box 'Flutters or quickening').

Week 21 and **week 22** are when you sense the first hints of uterine contractions. Your uterus has been contracting for many years now, but you are feeling it today because there is now enough pressure on your uterine muscles. Tightening of the uterus or contractions at this stage are typically painless. If there is pain, you need to speak to your doctor. Your uterus continues to grow and, by **week 23**, it is officially an abdominal organ.

Medical journals record an approximate 12 per cent women have 'nuchal cords' at **week 24** to **week 26** – with the numbers increasing closer to full term. Nuchal cord refers to when the umbilical cord gets wrapped around the baby's neck. Most of the time, this resolves itself before delivery. And even if it doesn't, it does not pose any impending threat in most cases. Your doctor will monitor this more closely through your subsequent ultrasounds.

'fundal length' in cm. Now, if this is your first pregnancy, this fundal length – give or take a couple of cm – sort of corresponds to the number of weeks you are pregnant. So, at 20 weeks, your fundal length will be roughly between 18 and 20 or 22 cm.

Is my baby growing?

This is possibly the *most* common fear among pregnant women in India. You're not alone in this. Has a family member scanned you from top to bottom, observed your abdomen and said something snide? Remember, it is perfectly normal for a lot of women to not show any signs of a growing bump till even five months of pregnancy. This is even more the case with women who have been fit before their pregnancy. It doesn't mean your baby is too small. Rely on your ultrasound and foetal measurements to gauge the growth of your baby. Nothing else matters except good old science.

Flutters or quickening

The very first butterfly 'flutter'-like foetal movements you will feel are termed 'quickening'. On an average, moms-to-be may first feel these hints of flutters from about 17 weeks of pregnancy to 20–25 weeks (even at 13 weeks, for second-time mums). It feels like gas, popping, bubbling, a growling tummy and/or butterflies in the stomach. Either way, remember each pregnancy is unique in its own way, and you may well feel your baby's movements earlier or later than this average too. It is your uterine muscle that senses these movements – not your abdominal muscle. There is no real pattern to these flutters, so you need not keep a track until trimester three, when many mums start counting kicks. If you haven't felt a single flutter till week 25, speak to your doctor about it.

By **week 25** and **week 26**, you should likely continue to gain the same amount of weekly weight. Your blood volume is now up by 25 per cent from week one of your pregnancy. Your fingers and ankles may swell because of this. Lower back pain can start around this time, as your shifting centre of gravity may be wearing down your abdominal muscles.

At **week 27**, your baby is getting pretty cramped in there, which means your uterus is expanding just a little bit more almost daily to accommodate your little one. Your lungs get a little cramped too, making you breathless. With your growing abdomen, your ribcage is also expanding! It is the lower ribcage that expands, not the upper. It will go back to its old size post pregnancy, though that doesn't always happen.

By **week 28**, you're wrapping up your sixth month of pregnancy. Globally, it has been observed that about 25 per cent babies are breech (i.e., head up and bottom down) at 28 weeks. At this point though, some babies are already positioned with their head down, their face looking to your back, chin tucked in and legs up. This is called the 'occipito-anterior position' and is the most ideal one for a normal vaginal delivery because it allows your baby to sail through your pelvis with more ease. Now is not the time to worry about your baby's position, though. Occipito-anterior or not, many things can change over the next three months.

What's your baby up to?

When I revisit my 3D and 4D ultrasound visuals now, it is almost creepy how much Taimur and Jeh look exactly like their sonos! It's creepy, and also lovely, I should add – to be able to glimpse at the life inside you with such clarity.

A QUICK END-OF-MONTH SUMMARY

Month 4

What's forming? Defined facial features, eyebrows, eyelashes; fine hair (called lanugo) and vernix (a wax-like coating) that protect her translucent skin

What's the end size? 4 to 5 inches (i.e., an elaichi banana)

What's the weight? Up to 0.19 kg

Month 5

What's forming? Muscles, ears, genitals, hair, eyelids, nerves, vocal chords; jerking, kicking, sipping, hiccuping reflexes; the heart rate evens out a little bit; cycles of sleep and wakefulness

What's the end size? 6 to 7 inches (i.e., an average money bill)

What's the weight? Up to 0.45 kg

Month 6

What's forming? Fat deposits; unique fingerprints; fully developed lungs; an ability to catch sounds from the outside; eyelids will open; reproductive organs; blood cells in the bone marrow

What's the end size? From 7 inches to a maximum of 12 inches (i.e., smaller than a foot-long ruler)

What's the weight? Up to 0.9 kg

Week 14: Your baby is beginning to swallow, taking super tiny sips of the amniotic fluid, which her kidneys then process into urine. Her neck is getting a little longer (and the ears are moving into their correct position at the sides of the head) and she has tiny little wrists and a chin. This is the stage where your baby can form meconium in her intestinal tract. This meconium stays in the tract through the pregnancy and usually comes out with her first poop post birth.

WHAT IS MECONIUM?

While growing in your uterus, your baby invariably absorbs many things: sips of amniotic fluid, bile from her liver, epithelial cells from her intestine, the lanugo (fine hair) from her skin, some mucus from the bowels. This is what forms into meconium that stays in your baby's body. It is basically your baby's poop – dark greenish-black and sticky.

Week 15: Your baby is the size of a pear and the little one can now hiccup! It won't be till much later in your pregnancy that you will feel the flutters when she hiccups, but it's easy to imagine. Your baby can now sense/hear little sounds from the outside world and your heartbeat. It isn't a silent temple inside your womb; remember that your baby is continuously exposed to the gentle and rhythmic sounds of your body. This is when your baby gets covered with lanugo.

Week 16: Your baby can flex and make fists, which means her nervous system and muscles are developing. She may attempt her first grab right now – the likeliest thing she will pull is the umbilical cord. Think of a lemon, if you're imagining her size (a lemon, mind you, not the Indian nimbu). Some 28 litres of blood is pumping through her circulatory system every day.

Week 17: Your baby's face is taking shape – this week she develops eyelashes, eyebrows and fingerprints! She is growing constantly and is developing her first formations of fat – so imagine that your little one is filling out slowly.

Week 18: Your 14 cm long baby can hear! You might feel her earliest movements now, as flutters mainly. If you could see your baby, she is likely to yawn or frown! That means her reflexes are developing. She is also oscillating between periods of sleep and wakefulness.

Week 19: Your baby is growing rapidly. You can imagine the little thing – a see-through bundle of nerves, vessels and organs (her skin is still transparent), almost like an *X-Men* of some sort! The lanugo may have by now covered your baby's head, shoulders and back. A fatty substance called myelin is also forming around your baby's nerves. This is what protects them and helps them make smoother movements as they grow up too. Remember the random grabs? Those may be turning into sturdy grips around now.

Week 20: As practice for her future feeds, your little one is sucking her thumb every so often. A white substance (like a layer of body lotion, of sorts) protects her skin in vitro. This is called vernix caseosa. This slippery coating will assist your baby's descent through the birth canal. It is amazing to imagine that, at this point, your baby girl's ovaries will already have millions of eggs and your baby boy's testes will begin to lower into the scrotum.

Week 21: If only you could look really close, you'd see the start of your baby's hair roots. She is now able to catch sounds from the outside, which means your voice and music. Your baby's gums are developing their second (permanent) set of teeth already. She is gaining fat and staying warm. The cartilage is hardening. The tiny, sensitive taste buds are developing. If you have multiple babies in your womb, they will become aware of each other around this time.

Week 22: After this stage, your baby will finally start weighing more than the placenta that she has been thriving on thus far. Her lungs are slowly developing – they will be the last organ to form fully. Right now, her oxygen is coming from your blood. Your baby's not quite breathing yet but she is practising to swallow. Her sensitivity to sounds is being honed now – on loud, jarring sounds. If someone advises you to lay off on watching a gory thriller on Netflix, this is where it's coming from! Your baby is developing taste buds, so she's probably getting a whiff of whatever you're eating. You never know how your appetite right now shapes your baby's reaction to new tastes in the future!

Week 23: Your baby has started her first low-impact kickboxing lesson – the jabs, kicks and rolls which may have begun gently a few weeks ago will be a little more pronounced. Someone who puts their hand to your belly may not yet be able to feel your baby move, but you are likely to. It may feel like a series of flutters. On the off chance you haven't felt a single movement yet (or up to week 25), you could speak to your doctor regarding your concerns.

Week 24: Your baby can raise her eyebrows, which means her facial muscles are working! The respiratory sacs in her lungs are multiplying right now. On an average, your baby is about 0.5 kg at this time – still lean but filling out.

Week 25: Your baby is peeing with regularity. Her digestive system has begun to show signs of the preliminary movements that aid digestion, even though there is no food in there yet. Her lungs are also developing at a steady pace. The hair on her head is actually white right now. The hair colour (pigment) is yet to form.

Week 26: She's curled up pretty cosily, but if you could hold your baby right now, she would quite likely be as long as your forearm (25–26 cm or so). Remember the eyes that were fused shut a long time ago? Well, those eyelids will be opening right about now. Her heart rate by now has slowed down somewhat, to about 140 beats per minute – but it's still faster than yours. Did you know a foetus has blue eyes at this stage? The colour of your baby's eye pigment begins to change only at the 31-week mark in vitro. Many babies' eyes develop into their true and final colour months after birth.

Week 27: The little one is sleeping and waking and has an active brain. Your baby's senses are developing really well and her eyes already display sensitivity to light. Now is the time people shine bright lights at their torsos, hoping to get the baby to move. She is now a super micro-sized version of what she will look like at birth. If you are having multiple babies, they have the same developmental milestones as a singleton. It is only at about 32 weeks that the growth of twins may begin to slow down a little (with triplets, the slowing down begins to happen at around 27–28 weeks) – this is pretty much because they're competing for the same resources.

Week 28: Your baby is sticking out her tongue, probably to taste the amniotic fluid. And her eyes are opening and shutting every so often – i.e., she is blinking. You know the REM (rapid eye movement) we experience when we're sleeping/dreaming? That's happening to your baby right now. The little one is really working on her sucking and breathing now, all in preparation for the real world. If she was born now, she would have a very good chance of survival.

(With inputs from Dr Mitossh Ruparel)

How will I feel: Symptoms of trimester two

I could party till 3 a.m. during Taimur's time, but I was in bed by 11 p.m. every single night during Jeh's time, except when I was shooting nights in Delhi. I couldn't keep my eyes open beyond 11 p.m.!

With your increasing energy levels of trimester two, you'll have a renewed sense of excitement. Your libido will kick into action, and sexual intercourse will be more tempting. You will want to travel. In fact, this is the time most parents-to-be opt to go for a 'babymoon'.

You may experience pain and sudden spasms from here on. As your belly grows, you may be dealing with **lower back pain** and aching joints. You may also feel sudden, jabbing pains on the sides of your stomach when you sleep. This is one of the most common problems during the later stages of pregnancy and is called **round ligament pain** (see section 'Round ligament pain'). Another common complaint well into trimester two is **headaches**. Usually, hydrating yourself, lying down and eating light will help.

Another highly inconvenient problem is **Symphysis Pubis**

Dysfunction (SPD). While your first instinct may be to panic, just remember to take a deep breath and assess your pain. SPD feels like a sharp needle-like pain in your pelvis (between your legs) and not like a uterine contraction or a menstrual type of cramp (see section 'Help! I have a sharp pain between my legs').

Towards the end of your second trimester, your baby is trying to settle into her birthing position. So imagine the double pressure of her head and your large uterus resting on your sciatic nerve, i.e., your lower spine. **Tingling, numbness, radiating or shooting pain** in your legs – any of these can happen.

You could also feel some **shortness of breath** because your uterus is starting to put pressure on your lungs. And you may even begin to snore! Your growing uterus may put pressure on your bladder as well, and you will possibly have accidental urine leakage, like when you cough, laugh or sneeze (see box 'I really need to pee a lot!'). Lastly, the additional volume of blood in your body will most likely make you feel **warm and sweaty**.

Eye irritation and vision distortion is common because the hormones are playing with the fluid build-up in your eyes. Be happy if your vision improves! However, if you feel the onset of more serious eye issues, run to your ophthalmologist.

Other symptoms could be nose bleeds, thrush, vaginal discharge (a clear/milky odourless discharge called leukorrhoea) and urinary tract infections (and let's not even get into **haemorrhoids**). Growing breasts, bleeding gums and the start of preliminary **Braxton-Hicks contractions** are not uncommon in the second trimester. Incidentally, Braxton-Hicks contractions are rare but not impossible in trimester two (see Chapter 3: Your Third Trimester). And **you may become clumsier**. Don't be alarmed to find yourself dropping things (see box 'Feeling clumsy and achy? Here's why').

It's good to bear in mind that a whole range of these symptoms (from swelling and abdominal pain to vaginal discharge and leaky nipples): (a) may or may not happen at all, (b) may happen early on from trimester two, (c) may show up well into trimester three.

Post the 16-week mark, you may start to **feel dizzy** getting up after having lain down in bed for a long time. Many moms find that they have to get out of bed slowly in the mornings because of the dizziness. Why is this? Simply put, the increasing hormones cause your blood vessels to widen and also relax, because of which there is increased blood flow to the baby (while the blood return to the mother is reduced).

This dizziness can happen any time through trimesters one to three. If the dizziness feels very pronounced, too frequent or out of the ordinary (light-headed, weak, sweaty, blurred vision, etc.), consult your doctor. Fluctuating blood sugar, blood pressure, anaemia or dehydration could be some of the other causes for dizziness (see box 'Anaemia: It's a lot more common than you'd think').

Reach for that moisturizer because your stretching skin may start feeling **itchy and dry**. A simple itchiness in your hands and feet is not uncommon, but be wary if it gets too intense – it might point to a liver disorder.

From this trimester on, you might experience a host of digestion- and eating-related side effects. You might be experiencing **acid reflux/heartburn** especially after meals because the hormones have relaxed your lower oesophageal sphincter (LES). You could try and manage those feelings of discomfort with smaller meal portions.

The **gag reflex** that first popped up in trimester one might still be going strong for a select few. This is a pharyngeal reflex, where you literally feel like gagging when something is put in your mouth (including large-sized foods or foods with unusual textures or any object like a dental tool or a toothbrush) or if you can smell something that feels unpleasant to you. You're gagging most likely because of the reflux.

While we are on the subject, a spot of **indigestion** is most likely par for the course. Why? While indigestion may first show up during your first trimester, owing to increasing hormones, it becomes more and more common during your second and third trimesters because your growing baby is basically pushing against your stomach. Add to that the fact that hormones are relaxing your muscles during pregnancy and therefore slowing down your digestion process too.

Constipation is another unfortunate side effect of most pregnancies. A high-fibre diet with a lot of fruits, nuts, eggs, seeds, water and vegetables is a great addition to the millets, grains and meats you have been eating already. And if it hasn't already happened, the bane of most pregnant women's existence – the awful haemorrhoids (simply put: piles) – may make an appearance too, although they are a lot more common in the third trimester.

Can you see swelling on your feet and fingers? That's **oedema**. What is oedema? With the whole churn of extra fluids and blood volume that your body is generating to develop your baby, your growing uterus is also putting pressure on your vena cava, which makes blood flow slow down at the legs. Your body's ability to expel water may also be lowered. All this adds up to oedema – simply put, swelling – in a pregnant woman's body. You might notice your fingers, hands, ankles or feet swell around this time. This is especially pronounced at the end of a long, tiring day or during hot weather or after excessive intake of salt or caffeine.

The swelling disappears on its own post delivery. It is scary when oedema is accompanied by weight gain, high blood pressure, dizziness, puffiness in the face, or if your hands and feet get excessively swollen. Very high oedema could indicate the onset of pre-eclampsia. Presence of proteins in your urine test will indicate the risk of pre-eclampsia.

Is there a 'pregnancy brain'?

I became pretty forgetful during my pregnancy. I noticed this a lot more during my second pregnancy and especially during the third trimester. I would randomly blank out. I would often be mid-conversation with Saif and would forget what I was talking about. I guess they call it the pregnancy stupids! I specifically remember the time we were in Dharamshala and I ordered a full dinner from in-room dining for Saif, Taimur and myself. Some 10 minutes later, I told Saif I needed to order dinner for us. I literally couldn't even recollect what my order was.

Pregnancy brain, placenta brain, mental mushiness or baby brain drain – it's got a lot of names and a fair amount of infamy, but don't worry about it. It is just a combination of hormone surges, exhaustion and sleeplessness that causes some (or all) things like forgetfulness, memory lapse, short attention span, lack of focus and/or short-term memory loss. It may creep up on you any time; trimesters don't matter here!

Let's take a deep dive into some of the more prominent issues of trimester two:

Round ligament pain

Your uterus is surrounded by a series of fibres that are holding it and connecting it to your pelvis. These fibres are the 'round ligament' that supports your belly through the pregnancy. When your uterus begins to grow, the round ligaments begin to pull at the nerves around it, and this can feel like a short, sharp stretching or stabbing sort of pain. You might feel it on one side or through your abdomen and even in your groin. The spasm hits especially when you roll over in bed, laugh, sneeze, cough, hiccup, stretch or move suddenly (like when getting out of bed or up from a chair). Don't worry; it's not harming your baby. Here are some things women do to ease their pains: (1) use a maternity belt for support, (2) try a gentle massage or mildly heated compresses, (3) improve posture, (4) sit down and breathe through the spasm, (5) use a wedge, or a U- or C-shaped pillow for support, (6) monitor physical activity, in case it is aggravating the pain.

Help! I have a sharp pain between my legs

Feel an excruciating pain when you turn sides in bed? Finding it impossible to put on a pair of trousers while standing up? It's Symphysis Pubis Dysfunction or SPD. Your pelvis comprises three bones that hold the uterus. The soft cartilage between the two bones that form the V-shape become significantly softer because of your pregnancy hormones. This occurs around the fifth month and carries on through the pregnancy. It feels like a sharp, piercing pain in your vagina and can be very scary. SPD can happen to anyone irrespective of age or weight. It is extremely common in Indian women.

Your SPD needs to be kept in check because you don't want your pelvis getting misaligned during the later stages of your pregnancy. Don't refrain from exercising; because inactivity will lead to other complications! Look for exercises to help with SPD and avoid certain postures. Icing your pelvic region helps. As does tying a scarf around your thighs and keeping your thighs glued together for 10 minutes, several times a day. Don't sit or stand with your legs wide apart. In fact, do avoid large steps and do take baby steps; the typical pregnancy 'waddling gait' is counterintuitive to SPD. Be careful when getting in and out of the car, i.e., keep your legs together.

Note: It is relevant to bear in mind that you may have pelvic girdle pain (PGP) at any point of time in your pregnancy. The SPD we discussed is one of the various pelvic pains that fall under the larger umbrella of PGP. Your pelvic girdle is basically the ring of bones that surrounds the base of your spine. So any pains in the front or back of your pelvis that affect your lower back, hips, groin or thighs can be PGP.

I REALLY NEED TO PEE A LOT!

Why does it happen: 1. The urge to urinate frequently starts at trimester one. Your pregnancy hormones have increased right from the first trimester as has the amount of blood flowing through your body. (2) These two things are making the blood flow to your kidneys quickly, which means your bladder fills up faster. (3) You're drinking a lot more water and other fluids during your pregnancy. (4) For the first 13 weeks or so your uterus is still a pelvic organ which is pressing down on your bladder, causing you to pee more frequently. Your urine frequency *may* normalize somewhat beyond 13 weeks, when your uterus moves up and becomes an abdominal organ.

How can you curb the frequency: (1) Limit your fluid intake from the evening, so your night sleep isn't disturbed. (2) Cut back on coffee, tea, soda (and alcohol!) – as these are all diuretics. (3) Keep doing your Kegels. (4) Here is a very handy tip throughout your pregnancy: Every time you go to pee, sit upright on the toilet seat and pee peacefully till your bladder feels completely empty. Breathe out. Count to 10. Lean forward a little bit to gently bend downwards. You will quite likely release a small second trickle of urine. Now your bladder is completely empty.

When is there something wrong: (1) If your urine is tinged with blood. (2) If you feel a burning sensation when you pee. (3) If you keep feeling the pressure of wanting to pee, but only a few drops come out. (4) If you feel discomfort in your abdominal and pelvic area. (5) If you have vaginal discharge. In these cases, speak to your doctor right away.

I get heartburn after every meal...

Acid reflux or heartburn is a harmless but a very uncomfortable burning sensation that pregnant women feel somewhere in their lower throat. This stems from indigestion, which is pretty common during pregnancy. Gas, bloating, indigestion, acid reflux – these are all interrelated issues. The hormones that are relaxing the muscles of your body (and your digestive process in the bargain) during pregnancy also end up 'relaxing' the valve – i.e., lower oesophageal sphincter – that separates your stomach and your oesophagus.

So, your gastric juices basically just seep upwards and cause a wicked burn in your throat. What can you do about it? Well, incorporate small, simple changes in your life to ease the heartburn: (1) wrap up dinner well before you sleep, (2) lie on your left side, (3) use a pillow to prop yourself up so you can keep the juices down, (4) eat smaller portions and chew your food well, (5) avoid acidic and sugary foods and beverages; eat a bowl of dahi, (6) take a short walk post meals.

Ugh! Why do I have haemorrhoids?

You can blame the progesterone in your body here. It basically starts relaxing the blood vessels in your rectum in preparation for birth while your baby is also pushing against these blood vessels as she grows bigger. Add to this the fact that many moms have a tendency towards constipation during this time, which means you are putting added pressure on your rectum. Imagine the haemorrhoid as a swollen varicose vein that is growing inside your anus (felt and not seen, and at times neither felt nor seen) or outside your anus (like a raised area or 'piles'). You may have difficulty and discomfort in using the toilet and may notice an itch, swelling, burn or bleed. Haemorrhoids are considered an embarrassing condition – well, don't let it faze you. Some 25 to 35 per cent pregnant women have them.

What can you do? (a) Keep up with your Kegels, (b) have lots of water and fibre-rich foods to keep your stool soft, (c) try a warm sitz bath (i.e., sit in a tub of warm water with salt and baking soda) or sit in a tub with plain warm water or warm water with Epsom salts, (d) use a doctor-prescribed, pregnancy-safe medicated ointment, (e) ice the area, uncomfortable as that sounds, (f) don't put pressure on your anus, so sleep on your side, walk around rather than sit and use an inflatable ring to sit on. If it's bad enough to require medical intervention, go with your doctor's advice.

My lower back hurts

I really worked hard during my pregnancies. And during Jeh's time, I was 40, I was living through a pandemic, moving homes and working. I had intense pain in my lower back. I didn't get any massages though.

This is possibly one of the most common pains during pregnancy and most often radiates from the sacroiliac joint in your lower back. This is the joint that connects the two bones of the pelvis with strong ligaments and helps support your upper body weight. Because of its strategic location, this joint faces a great deal of pressure from your growing uterus, your increasing weight and when you change posture. What can you do? Not much, except exercises that bring you relief (under the guidance of a doctor, prenatal specialist, fitness trainer, chiropractor or physiotherapist). Use cold fomentation/ice packs and warm packs on the area. Pop a pregnancy-safe painkiller and beg your partner to give you a nightly back rub! Remember, your uterus has moved from your pelvis (low) into your abdomen (high), and your ligaments have loosened with pregnancy hormones. Please note that if your lower back pain is accompanied by tingling sensations or a radiating pain going till the legs or a sudden change in your urine/stool patterns – call your doctor.

A BACK RUB AT THE END OF A LONG DAY

Saif gives the best foot massages! Because he loves getting foot massages more than anything else, he has actually mastered the art of giving the best ones. I, for one, was very thankful for that! And he was always there for me whenever I was tired, unnerved or just down, or if dealing with Taimur was getting on my nerves (it happens to all of us!). He may not write romantic notes on Instagram or give gushy interviews about his wife, but Saif had a knack for balancing everything out. 'I'll sort it out,' are his words, always.

A back rub helps in relaxing and soothing those aching muscles. If you cannot or do not want to arrange for an appointment with a qualified neonatal massage therapist, you could always ask your partner, mom or friend to give you one. A few key points to bear in mind are: (a) stick to gentle oils or moisturizing creams that will not cause any allergic reactions, (b) lie on your side and use pillows to support your legs, (c) keep the strokes smooth and long and gentle, while working downwards from the neck, (d) don't press any points on the wrist, knuckles, ankles, feet or palms, or have massages given directly on the spine, (e) look up a home pregnancy massage video from a reliable site to see how the hands must be positioned (knuckle, fist or palm massage) and which direction to massage in (i.e., away from the spine).

FEELING CLUMSY AND ACHY? HERE'S WHY

You should know by now that your body has been taken over by hormones! You've learnt all about hCG, progesterone and oestrogen. Now say hello to relaxin. This hormone, along with progesterone, helps to relax, widen and soften your pelvis and cervix to prepare you for giving birth. On the flip side, it can loosen your ligaments and joints. It is this possible 'relaxation' of your hands, fingers and wrists that may make you feel like you have butterfingers.

Your centre of gravity is also shifting as your stomach grows, which could make you feel unbalanced. The 'don't wear heels' advice you'll hear stems from this. You might also feel achy. The fluid retention in your body is very high right now (blood volume too), so there is more pressure on all your blood vessels. In tight spaces of your body (like the carpal tunnel of the wrist), such swelling can cause nerves to compress, making you feel achy.

How will I look?

Through both my pregnancies I watched my body change and I didn't care. Sure, I was used to being a certain body type but when I couldn't put on that pair of jeans, I Instagrammed it. When I wore a sexy gown, I Instagrammed that too.

Some moms look and feel sexy at this stage in their pregnancy. While your waistline may begin to disappear, your body will have a new topography of curves. Enjoy it! Remember that on an average, you'll gain weight at the rate of half a kilo per month.

Of course these assumptions change if you are carrying multiple babies and also if you have a predisposition to gain weight.

If you have an average, healthy pregnancy during which you are physically active, **you can possibly expect anywhere from a 2.5 to 6.5 kg range of weight gain** in your second trimester. However, **a maximum of 9 kg** is acceptable, especially if you have been underweight before your pregnancy and the rest of your health parameters (like blood sugar and blood pressure) are normal. For women who have been overweight prior to their pregnancy and for women with diabetes, the doctor usually runs a really tight ship and tries to keep the weight gain within the 5 to 6 kg zone.

Your belly button ('innie') may suddenly just pop out ('outie') – it will retreat again post baby. You may be showing fairly by now. Some women tend to get conscious about their growing bump and often develop an involuntary slouch during this time – it's an easy habit to get out of, if you remain mindful of the tendency.

Your breasts may begin to grow as will the areolas (the pigmented portion around the nipples), which may also get darker. It is the normal flux of hormones and blood volume that is affecting the glands and tissues of your breasts. Alongside this comes an increase of fat deposits – which is a precursor to lactation. Many pregnant women also notice small bumps on their areolas. These are nothing but your skin's oil (or sebaceous) glands, which usually become prominent during a menstrual cycle or during pregnancy. These bumps even have an official name: Montgomery's tubercles! If you notice any discharge from your nipples, change in breast shape, dimpled skin on the breast, a swelling of a lymph node in the armpit or a breast lump – tell your doctor about it right away.

With your growing bump, you may notice a host of changes in your skin in trimester two. As we've said before, some of you may have that pregnancy glow (or an attractive flush) while others will grapple with pregnancy acne. Your dry skin may turn oily or vice versa. You may suddenly find darkened patches of pigmentation in different areas of your body (most commonly the back of the neck, thighs and underarms) and on your face. It is perfectly normal and there is nothing you can do about it (see Chapter 10: Self-Care).

Don't get stressed if many of you see the sudden appearance of stretch marks on your stomach, thighs, breasts or buttocks. If you have an unholy fear of stretch marks, just breathe! It is par for the course if you have a genetic predisposition to it. You will be helpless as those lines start appearing on your belly – in varying colours, right from red, pink, brown, purple or a blend of these. You may even remain stretch mark free till the last week of your pregnancy – and then suddenly find those annoying lines all across your stomach!

Your hormones are in overdrive and can easily be blamed for all that is happening to you – good and bad. You can easily choose to tackle all these cosmetic hiccups at leisure, after you have had your baby (see Chapter 10: Self-Care). Late into trimester two, spider veins and/or varicose veins may make their debut. While not every pregnant woman has this, the linea nigra makes its appearance gradually from here on. It is a distinctly dark line (1 cm wide hyperpigmentation) going vertically up the centre of your abdomen. Why does the linea nigra form? Blame it on your hormones!

But it's not all stretch marks and weight gain. Many of you will now enjoy lush hair. Your pregnancy growth hormones are holding on to all those strands that we shed daily in the routine course of things, giving you a lovely head full of hair.

My skin is going nuts: Stretch marks, spider veins, varicose veins, skin darkening

Let's break these down simply as some or all of these can happen to many women during their second and last trimesters.

Stretch marks: If you are genetically predisposed to stretch marks (check your mom, grandmom or aunt for stretch marks), you will find it is unavoidable. The only difference is when it starts! Stretch marks depend on the inherent elasticity of your skin. You can moisturize yourself well to avoid itchiness and dry skin though.

Spider veins and varicose veins: The increasing blood flow places pressure on your vessels and causes tiny red veins to form on your skin. These are spider veins and will fade away post delivery. Varicose veins, on the other hand, are different. Your growing abdomen and weight can put pressure on your legs and constrict blood flow (imagine a bottleneck) to your lower body. The veins of your legs turn purplish/blue – the colour of a bruise. It is a cosmetic inconvenience. Varicose veins take longer to fade post delivery and may need medical intervention.

Skin darkening: You will find velvety dark or black patches commonly at the back of your neck, in your underarms and between your thighs. This is acanthosis and is a reaction in your body to hormones, weight gain, insulin resistance and metabolic change. Apart from acanthosis, sun sensitivity combined with oestrogen and progesterone can be responsible for melasma (aka chloasma) – dark brown patches on the forehead, cheeks, nose or chin. Such hyperpigmentation is not harmful. Address it post pregnancy (see Chapter 10: Self-Care).

Your emotions

I was in a very different zone through my second pregnancy and had a rough time with low blood pressure and exhaustion. I tried hard and kept up with my professional commitments but I have to admit I couldn't have done anything without Saif's continuous support and Taimur's love. I relied heavily on the two of them! Saif is always just a phone call away from me, whether he is away shooting or I am. I know that he has my back and that really is the biggest reassurance for me. Every evening, Saif would be the one to say, 'What do you want to do', 'What do you feel like eating', 'Which movie do you want to watch'. He creates a very warm and loving family atmosphere for Taimur and me. And he gives me a foundation to stand on. He was always there for Taimur, completely hands-on. I never felt, even for a second, that I was doing this on my own.

You are likely to begin this trimester with a sort of renewed zeal. The first trimester anxieties are gone. The baby is still a few months away. You will be feeling energetic and ready to enjoy this phase of your pregnancy. It could be a great feeling to have your libido back. Increased blood flow to your pelvic region can enhance your sex drive. Rediscovering intimacy can be a very positive experience for you at this point. But do remember – at any point of time in your pregnancy – you may not feel the same way as another pregnant woman. And that is absolutely fine.

For many mothers, it's the second trimester when it all becomes 'real'. With it may come certain fears especially if you are a first-time mom. Many moms worry about the labour and its pain. First-time moms also stress about breastfeeding their child and whether they can manage it. You might also be planning some changes to your home, thinking of a baby room and buying other home-related products to make this transition in life smoother. It is a good idea to plan ahead.

This is a great time to address the upcoming addition to your family with your partner and your extended family. Think about the things that matter. Where and how you want to give birth: Do you have a birthing plan; do you want a birthing plan? Do you need an additional set of hands to help you with your baby: will it be a maid, a nurse or a specialized baby maid (commonly called a jhappa maid); do you want to do this on your own? (P.S.: Any good Indian paediatrician will advise you to – at the very outset – assert your authority so your helper and your family are clear that your baby will be looked after as per your wishes and your protocol! This advice has held many moms in good stead.)

How do you want your baby to be looked after: what roles will your family members play? How will you accommodate this baby in your life? You can start to plan a nursery for your baby. If you don't have a dedicated nursery or bedroom for your baby, how will you plan the space? Even a simple thing like making a shopping list that you can execute later will help (see Part III: Getting Ready for the Baby: Your Definitive Guide to Shopping and Planning for the Nursery). Think about when you should and could return to work and how to manage it.

You can start working on your common, upcoming-third-trimester anxieties from now, by speaking to your doctor, family and friends about childbirth or joining a prenatal class (if available) that will help you navigate labour, post-delivery self-care, childcare and breastfeeding. You would much rather be overprepared than underconfident.

WHAT DO PEOPLE EXPECT? WHAT DO I EXPECT?

With Sonali Gupta, clinical psychologist

While two people make a choice to get married, it's important to remember that in India people get married into a family. The same holds true for a baby. A baby is part of the larger ecosystem, and, as a result, pregnancy maybe the time where everyone right from your mother or mother-in-law and even extended family may have advice for you that they may want you to follow. This can be daunting and tricky to navigate.

- Allow yourself to be: Should you pen a list of goals on what you expect from your nine months? For a lot of women, task lists leave them anxious and exhausted. Post delivery, there will be enough things to focus on and 'do'. Use your pregnancy to experience 'being' and enjoy this beautiful phase. Build realistic expectations, even from your own self.

- Very often, it is during pregnancy that women find themselves inundated with advice in relation to rituals and even superstitions or beliefs around pregnancy and childbirth. It may be important to learn when to listen and yet not react, when to filter the feedback on your own, and when to be assertive. Also learn to discuss pertinent topics with your partner or gynaecologist and buy time before commenting on some issues.

- The money talk: Do a financial check. Where are you placed? How much do you spend? Sometimes people overspend, and at other times people overthink. Both are equally dangerous. There will be a ton of things you may want to buy that your baby will not even need. Don't stretch yourself financially. It's okay to have a conversation about money and your baby's needs, and reach a decision mindfully.

- Do your research: Your pregnancy is a great time to gather your resources and do your research. Typically, many Indian families tend to be very involved in the life of a new mom and her baby. And while it is wonderful to have the social support, sometimes you and your family may have differing ideas about child rearing. Here are examples of some issues where very often I see clients and their families struggle. It could be anything from breastfeeding and bottle feeding to a postnatal massage. What if you don't want that maalish? Where are you going to have the baby? What will your first 40 days look like? Opening these conversations allows people to build realistic expectations and also understand what you and your partner have in mind.

- Keep talking: Communicate with your partner, parents and/or in-laws on what life will look like post having the baby. What if your mother on whom you were relying is unable or unwilling to give you a hand? Having a conversation on roles and responsibilities in advance gives you enough time to weigh your options and even plan to some degree.

What am I allowed to do?

Kareena was sick through a large chunk of her second pregnancy. We were in the middle of the pandemic, and she went to Delhi to do night shoots in her second trimester. I was in tears every day. I would wait for her to call me on her way home after her shoot. I didn't want to show her my anxiety but I knew how tough it was for her. When she came back to Mumbai, she told me how there were 300 people around her and she shot in rickshaws. I don't know how I would have felt if I had known that while she was away. I am definitely a more cautious and conservative person. I often reprimanded her during both her pregnancies: for working too hard or partying too hard. But her zest and determination for life are inspirational. I have true respect for her. She has been so strong through her pregnancies and has set the bar so high for many women out there. She was completely nonchalant about the fact that she was a pregnant working woman and she had her own set of responsibilities. Her work gives her joy, and she always does things her way. Finishing her tasks is what keeps her ticking. She has been focused and creative through both her pregnancies, and I know both her babies definitely felt that.
— KARISMA KAPOOR, sister

You can actually do whatever you set your mind to, as long as your doctor is confident and you are happy. You're in the easiest zone of your pregnancy at this point of time. If you have a delicate pregnancy, there will be restrictions involved.

REASONS YOU MAY END UP ON BED REST

It is not uncommon for a few of you to end up on bed rest during any of your trimesters for short durations of time. Bed rests can vary between scheduled hours of rest per day, strict and complete bed rest, hospitalized bed rest or bed rest with allowances.

A possible complication midway through your pregnancy can put you on bed rest till the end of term too. In certain pregnancies, a woman may even be on bed rest for the whole nine months. There is a list of reasons and complications that may lead your doctor to put you on bed rest. Some of the causes may be:

- Placenta complications (like placenta previa, etc.)
- Cervical incompetence and/or short cervix – thereby risking premature labour or preterm delivery
- Vaginal bleeding
- A precious pregnancy and/or a history of repeated miscarriage or stillbirth
- High blood pressure; pre-eclampsia; pregnancy-induced hypertension
- IVF moms with obstetric complications like a risk of preterm labour on account of twins, shortened cervix or a previous history of preterm birth

However, **staying physically active in your pregnancy is extremely important,** so always take the time to understand why you have ended up on bed rest. Bed rest comes with its disadvantages, and clinical evidence has not always reflected an improved birth outcome. Lack of movement can cause blood clots to form (especially in the legs) – this is known as deep vein thrombosis. Women tend to get depressed, stressed or anxious because they're in bed all day, they're feeling dependent on other people, and/or they cannot go to work. Prolonged periods in bed can also cause a loss in muscle conditioning along with body ache and lower back pain. It is, in general, detrimental to pregnant women.

Can I get a massage?

Massages are not advisable in the early part of your first trimester, but prenatal massages can be a wonderful way to relax and ease those aching limbs in this middle phase of your pregnancy. Always, always pick a therapist or expert who is trained for prenatal massages or go to reputed spas that offer prenatal massages. At this stage, not all oils will be suitable for you. Do be careful. Certain massage techniques, such as acupressure, could lead to uterine contractions, so you need a trained therapist. Don't be scared, just be careful. It's also lovely to get a back rub from your partner or a family member as you get more and more achy (see box 'A back rub at the end of a long day'). There are a lot of easy pregnancy massage videos online for them to follow, but do get it checked and cleared by your doctor.

Can I have sex?

Your first trimester fears about hurting your baby are hopefully gone by now. A penis cannot penetrate deep enough to knock your baby on the head, nor can your baby tell what's going on! The sensitivity in your cervix, which may have caused post-intercourse bleeds, might also have eased. Your energy levels are high, and the blood flow to your pelvis has quite likely gotten your libido back. However, your belly has grown into a proper bump, and you may feel sensitive in your genitals or on your breasts. This could make things tougher.

You will not be able to engage in the missionary position or lie on your stomach through your pregnancy. Find positions to harbour your growing belly without scaring you – like lying on the side facing each other, a spooning position, standing, you on top, reverse cowgirl or getting on your fours. Sex toys and aides are also safe, as long as it's good quality and kept very clean (check with your doctor, though, if you have any pregnancy complications).

Remember, it is also okay to not want to engage in any sexual activity. You can definitely find other ways and means to connect with your partner intimately (see section 'Your emotions'). Again, oral sex is also safe; but it is advisable to not blow air directly into the vagina. Why? Although it is very rare, research shares that it can potentially cause an air embolism. If your partner has an active STD or has been recently diagnosed with one, avoid sex completely.

Exercise

Refer to the exercise tips shared in trimester one. Remember, your fitness routines shouldn't make you breathless. And, like you were doing earlier, follow your doctor's advice on racquet sports, extremely jumpy moves or routines that could potentially make you susceptible to falls. Continue doing what you have always been doing pre-pregnancy. Do consult your doctor at all stages.

Midway through trimester two, you might find running is tougher. It's the hormone relaxin at play that may be loosening your ligaments. You can start on a course of internationally accredited prenatal exercises on your own or through a good local prenatal instructor. These movements won't just help for the remainder of your six months but may also assist in a smoother delivery. More than anything else, it will help you get back on your feet (and regain strength) faster post baby. Any fitness routine you follow diligently will help too!

Yoga asanas that help you stretch your pelvis and maintain your back strength are great. Swimming is a good exercise. Incorporate a few minutes of Kegels multiple times a day, every day. If you're home-bound, keep up your momentum by doing a short sequence of gentle movements where you wiggle your toes, circle your ankles and arms and try to bend and touch your toes gently. Try a few side bends, pelvic raises, twists, the cat and cow pose, butterfly flaps and other such simple stretches.

GETTING YOUR KEGELS DONE

Kegel exercises are meant to strengthen the muscles of your pelvic floor. The simplest form is contracting and relaxing your pelvic muscles – like trying to stop the flow of urine midstream. You can do this any time, anywhere. Try right now! It is ideal to do this for a few minutes every day, two to five times a day. Just sit comfortably and squeeze and hold (for five seconds) and then release (for five seconds) your pelvic muscles for 10–15 counts. Alternate it with 10–15 rapid squeeze-and-release counts. The advantages of keeping up with your Kegels from early on in your pregnancy are: (a) improved bladder and bowel control, (b) preventing urinary incontinence, (c) pushing during labour, (d) better pelvis recovery post childbirth, (e) lowering the risk of vaginal prolapse. Join a prenatal class or use a book or website to visualize different postures for Kegels. You can sit on a chair, squat, use a Kegel ball, do wall sits, lie on your back and thrust your hips up, sit in the butterfly pose or be on your fours.

Eating

I am not a follower of superfoods. Raw foods and juices don't suit my body, and I would rather have a bowl of hot mutton paya soup any day! I would say – eat the right stuff. I would often give in to my cravings but then compensate by eating right for the next 48 hours.

You don't need to eat lots more in terms of your caloric intake. Instead focus on eating better (see box 'Do I need to eat more?'). The same food rules that we discussed in trimester one apply throughout your pregnancy. Be mindful of your proteins and fibre. And definitely add millets to your diet: this is a great pregnancy and post-pregnancy tip. The most common millets in India are jowar (sorghum), bajra (pearl), ragi (finger), barri (common), kangni (foxtail), kodra (kodo) and jhangora (barnyard).

Many Indian women have anaemia and iron deficiency even in the routine course of things, more so during pregnancy. It is easy to get caught up with lists of high iron, high folate or high calcium foods. But what is actually critically important is the assimilation of nutrition in your body (see Chapter 8: Nutrition).

Feel like having that slice of pineapple or a small bowl of papaya? Please do. There are fears surrounding certain fruits or vegetables being pregnancy 'unsafe' – like papaya, pineapple and grapes and moringa, radish, excess potatoes, eggplant and moong bean sprouts. As long as you're not having a football-sized serving, anything in moderation is fine. Indulge your cravings; now is the time to do so. But just remember before you polish off that chocolate cake, your baby needs wholesome nutrition, which she can only take from your body!

Why do I have cravings?

Feel like peanut butter with dosa? How about a packet of Lays chips crushed on top of your noodles? Pineapple pizza for breakfast? Pickles with ice cream or rotis with Nutella. A pregnancy craving is precisely that – a desperate urge to consume something, often out of the ordinary (and very often not a regular go-to food item for you). It is very common. On an average, pregnancy cravings commence during the first trimester – around the time you may begin symptoms of morning sickness. The cravings really spike during the second trimester. Thereafter, they ease off during the third trimester. But this is on an average! Don't worry if you have a different pattern.

You remember reading about how all those hormonal fluctuations affect your appetite, and play with your sense of taste and smell? That could be one cause for cravings. A sort of desire to feel a different texture on your palette. Nutritionists say a craving is also a signal from your body, a signal to feed it something it wants: say, for instance, calcium or iron or carbohydrates. It could stem from stress – cravings are your comfort foods. Don't forget your body also needs more energy at this time. A craving is not always sugar: pregnant women are known to crave everything from red meat, pickles and pasta, to potatoes, ice cream or hot chillies.

Note: Don't be surprised if you develop another extreme, i.e., aversion to certain foods, smells, tastes and textures.

Do I need to eat more?

My appetite increased tangibly every trimester. I know there are many moms who don't gain any weight during pregnancy, but my body is different. Through both my pregnancies, I was absolutely comfortable with the amount of weight I gained. I think I overdid things in my first pregnancy and really piled on the calories. I was excited and didn't care. Everyone has to fall off the wagon every so often. I noticed a significant increase in appetite during my second trimester during both pregnancies though.

Feeling hungry? It is perfectly normal. After the nausea and morning sickness of trimester one, where you may not have felt like eating, your second trimester will quite likely renew your appetite. You may feel especially hungry when you wake up in the morning or during the course of the night. It is simply because you're going longer hours without a meal. Your baby is growing and demanding more nourishment from you.

If you were to really break it down, the global average says your body needs an extra 300–350 calories per day in the second trimester and an extra 500 calories per day in the third trimester. This is compared to what you were eating before you conceived. However, the rules and regulations of your pregnancy nutrition will always vary if, say, you were overweight before pregnancy, if you have blood sugar and blood pressure issues during pregnancy, if you're carrying multiple babies, if you're on bed rest or are physically active, and so forth.

> Here's a quick tip: Eating smaller meals more frequently may help stabilize your blood sugar, keep you full and aid with digestive or reflux issues too. Carry small snacks with you when you leave your house because a hunger pang can hit you at any time. Snack ideas? Dates, dried figs, mixed nuts, a fresh fruit, a bottle of fresh lime water or soda and a bottle of water.

Can I travel?

If you are a first-time mom, this kid-free/chaos-free time is never coming back. Culturally, we tend to have a fair amount of superstitions surrounding the first trimester of pregnancy – the big one being to stay in and stay safe. But the second trimester is a lot more carefree. Speak to your doctor and have him/her clear you to travel. Usually your doctor will have you do an ultrasound before you leave and soon after you come back, for precaution – especially if it's a trip which involves long hours of travelling. As with your first trimester, you may be put on a couple of additional medicine supplements by your doctor. For a long flight, carry compression socks if you're hypercoagulable. Follow the same travel advice as shared in trimester one closely.

What can't I do?

Stick to the same don'ts as discussed in trimester one. Keep a close watch on your caffeine and alcohol intake. Much like you did from the start of your pregnancy, continue to avoid X-rays and hot tubs/saunas.

BE CAREFUL IN THE BATHROOM

No, this isn't some random advice! Being careful in the bathroom is very important when you're pregnant. There are multiple reasons that have prompted this list:

- Don't use very hot water for your baths. It can make you feel dizzy or light-headed.
- Install a handle if you're stepping in and out of a tub for your showers: basically, recee your bathroom – can you slip and fall if the floor is wet or soapy? You cannot be falling during pregnancy.
- When you pee, always wipe and dry your genitals. Be very careful to wash/wipe from front to back after using the toilet. You have to stay as safe as possible to prevent UTIs or other infections.
- In public bathrooms, avoid sitting on the toilet seat. If that is impossible, carry wet wipes, a toilet seat sanitizing spray and a disposable toilet seat cover with you.
- While we're at it, look after your oral hygiene with utmost diligence. Dental and oral issues are not uncommon during pregnancy.

What happens at the doctor's?

Being pregnant during a pandemic was worrisome, but I relied completely on my doctor's guidance. I did every scan and test by the book. I am very thorough, very professional – a real Virgo. Despite my work schedule, I didn't skip a single doctor's visit or ultrasound appointment. I asked them lots of questions. Was my baby's weight right? Was my weight gain okay? I would barrage my sonologist with questions with half an eye on the 4D scanner so I could see what my baby looked like.

Your doctor will see you every two to four weeks during your second trimester. This trimester, you'll go through some of the key ultrasounds and blood tests. You will be scanned for birth defects and will undergo other genetic screening tests. You will also be given vaccines during these three months and will undergo a diabetes test.

What tests and vaccines will I need to take?

1. **Blood tests**

   Here is the blood test list that is prescribed in trimester two:
   - **16 weeks**: Quadruple marker test – it helps in evaluating whether there are increased chances of Down syndrome, spina bifida (neural tube defects), trisomy 18 or abdominal wall defects in the foetus. It can be done up till 22 weeks of pregnancy too. The 'quad' screen measures 'four' substances in a pregnant woman's blood: (1) alpha-fetoprotein (AFP) made by your baby; (2) hCG hormone made by your placenta; (3) estriol hormone made by your placenta and your baby's liver; (4) inhibin A hormone, again, made by your placenta. If you have done an NIPT earlier in your pregnancy with satisfactory results your doctor might skip this one.
   - **26–28 weeks**: Depending on your doctor, you will be asked to undergo these blood tests between 26 weeks (end of trimester two) and 28 weeks (early in trimester three):

a. HbA1C and blood sugar fasting – this is to keep a close check on your blood sugar levels

b. Oral GTT (glucose tolerance test) – i.e., 'diabetes test', done at 24 to 28 weeks. This test evaluates the ability of your body to absorb specific amounts of glucose. It entails fasting blood glucose followed by 75 grams oral glucose solution and then two hours post-glucose levels. This test is not repeated again unless there is a suspicion of late onset of gestational diabetes due to polyhydramnios or a very big baby

c. CBC – for haemoglobin levels

d. Iron studies – a complete study of iron, ferritin and transferrin – if the CBC test listed above indicates anaemia

e. FT3, FT4, TSH – for thyroid

2. **Urine test**
26–28 weeks: Again, depending on your doctor, you will be asked to undergo a urine test between 26 weeks (end of trimester two) and 28 weeks (early in trimester three). Urine tests during your pregnancy are completely harmless and also essential. What are these pregnancy urine tests doing for you? (1) Detecting proteins like albumin in your urine that could be a sign of pregnancy-induced hypertension, toxemia or pre-eclampsia. (2) Detecting glucose or sugars in your urine that may indicate gestational diabetes or pre-existing diabetes. (3) Detecting RBCs or WBCs that can indicate UTIs.

3. **Vaccines***
Tetanus Toxoid (TT): Two doses of TT at least 28 days apart to be given to all pregnant women commencing from

---

* As per FOGSI recommendations

the second trimester. If a subsequent pregnancy occurs within five years, only one booster is given

Flu vaccine: After 26 weeks; or at any time if there is an ongoing pandemic

Tdap vaccine: For tetanus, diphtheria, whooping cough (pertussis), between 28 and 36 weeks

A breakdown of your second trimester ultrasounds

Two tests are important for all pregnant women at this time. If you're having an IVF baby or multiple babies, you could possibly have at the least one additional routine ultrasound in the second trimester. While your placenta is examined at each ultrasound, importance is given to cervical measurements especially for older mums and mums with twins – to estimate preterm birth (see box 'Why are cervical measurements useful?').

- **At 16 weeks**: An ultrasound report to accompany the quadruple marker blood test – though this isn't always par for the course. This test becomes mandatory when the first trimester screening indicates a higher risk of possible genetic disease, or in case of multiple pregnancies.
- **At 18–20 weeks**: Anomaly scan to rule out any abnormalities (see box 'Why is the 18–20-week anomaly scan so important?'). It is perfectly normal to feel a little nervous about this scan. After all, it's the big one where your baby is measured and examined for a whole host of things. Many parents-to-be (and grandparents-to-be) also tend to be excited about this scan. Your baby is fully formed by now! You can see your baby's hands, fingers, legs, feet, spine and face. You can see the shape of her head, and you'll catch a glimpse of what

the little one's up to in there. You may just catch your baby sucking her thumb, kicking, wriggling or trying to make a grab at something. You are also pretty much midway through your pregnancy, which makes it fun to figure out your baby's weight. You'll also be amazed at how much you can tell from a 3D/4D scan of your little one – just so long as she has decided to position just right!

Quick tip: Most ultrasounds will require a full bladder. So stay prepared in advance and up your fluid intake, so your sonologist doesn't end up making you wait as you sip on that one-litre bottle of water to fill up your bladder! Drink about two to three glasses of water an hour prior to your scheduled appointment and do not pass urine. You needn't be bursting full! In fact, drinking two to three litres is going to make you feel pukey and uncomfortable. A full bladder is excruciating by the time your scan ends, though. Scope out the nearest toilet, is the best advice here!

WHY IS THE 18–20-WEEK ANOMALY SCAN SO IMPORTANT?

This is probably the most detailed ultrasound of your entire pregnancy. Here is what is being looked at and measured: your baby's size, face, brain, spine, heart and heart rate, kidneys, diaphragm, chest, stomach, bladder, genitals, limbs – all this is examined for structural abnormalities. Plus, the umbilical cord, amniotic fluid level, placenta location and cervix (to see if it is closed and long) are all checked.

With this test, the sonologist is scanning your foetus for markers of **genetic/chromosomal disorders** such as Down syndrome and trisomy 18. If this screening indicates a high risk for chromosomal anomalies in the foetus, then you will be asked to undergo one or both invasive tests that detect abnormalities:

(1) CVS or chorionic villus sampling (where a catheter or needle is used to biopsy placental cells)
(2) Amniocentesis (where a small sample of the amniotic fluid that surrounds the foetus is removed and examined)

From these samples, the cells of the foetus are isolated from the placental tissue and the amniotic fluid, and cultured in a genetic lab. They are then examined for the structure of all the 46 chromosomes. This process is called karyotyping, and a report of this analysis takes two to three weeks. Both these procedures are as such 'minor' ones done on an outpatient basis (i.e., you don't need to be hospitalized). However, since these procedures are invasive in nature, they carry a small risk of miscarriage and vaginal bleeding. These procedures are performed by a sonologist, who is specially trained and experienced in conducting these tests and can explain all the risks and benefits involved.

Note: Many mums who have conceived at an older age – for the sake of abundant precaution – voluntarily opt for invasive tests like CVS or amniocentesis because it is generally believed that babies born to older women have a higher risk of chromosomal conditions. And these two diagnostic procedures have an almost complete accuracy rate.

> *NIPS or NIPT ideally done at 10 weeks of pregnancy – that we discussed in the first trimester – will play an important role in determining the course of action your doctor will prescribe vis-à-vis amniocentesis or CVS.*
>
> **(With inputs from Dr Mitossh Ruparel)**

- **At 23 weeks**: Your sonologist may recommend one more anomaly scan along with a cardiac scan of your baby. (This may be a good time to squeeze in that 3D/4D scan.)

If you want that one good 3D/4D scan through your entire pregnancy, then pick the earlier part of your 20- to 30-week phase for it. A good 4D image depends on the position of the foetus, how much it's moving and the volume of the surrounding fluid. While your baby has visible features for you to see post 28 weeks, the in vitro visibility may be less if the foetus is in an unfavourable position. If you scan too early, you may not get a good look at your baby's features. – DR MITOSSH RUPAREL, sonologist

WHY ARE CERVICAL MEASUREMENTS USEFUL?

Your cervix is the closed, long and firm cylindrical portion that connects your uterus with your vagina. It shortens and softens slowly in the course of your pregnancy. It stays closed to keep the baby in. The cervix is usually 30 to 50 mm long during pregnancy. Some women have a naturally shorter cervix. And if during pregnancy the cervix becomes too short too soon, there's a risk of miscarriage or premature birth. If your cervix is less than approximately 25 mm towards the tail end of your second trimester, it is considered a 'short cervix'.

A short cervix is also caused by something called an incompetent (or insufficient) cervix. The pressure of the growing baby presses on the cervix. If 'short', the cervix opens up before the baby is ready to birth. It could potentially be a cause for miscarriage. If you feel an onset of pelvic pressure, abdominal cramps, backache, Braxton-Hicks contractions, vaginal discharge or spotting, you could possibly have a short cervix. You absolutely have to rely on your ob-gyn to guide you through this issue. He/She could prescribe strict bed rest, a cervical stitch, supplemental progesterone or other treatment plans.

Note: By rule of thumb, your sonologist will closely monitor your cervical length measurement if you're carrying multiple babies – whether through IVF or conceived naturally.

(With inputs from Dr Mitossh Ruparel)

What medicines do I need?

The good thing is, you're most likely to be feeling your best. Continue your prenatal vitamins religiously. And always check prescription drugs and supplements with your doctor before consuming anything. Refer to the tips shared in trimester one for pregnancy medicines. All pregnant women in India are given iron and calcium supplements from the second trimester till the end of term. This is to prevent iron-deficiency anaemia and depleting calcium levels in the mother – a natural occurrence with the growing demands of a baby on the body. Some women may need protein supplements in addition.

Complications of trimester two

Bleeding, much like in trimester one, will be a cause of worry at any stage in your pregnancy. The onset of **pregnancy-induced hypertension** and **pre-eclampsia** because of blood pressure as well as **gestational diabetes** because of blood sugar are all red flags.

Your second trimester is also the only time a **Medical Termination of Pregnancy (MTP)** is possible, if required for any reason. It is also described as an induced abortion and is legally permissible and medically safe up to 24 weeks of gestation. Depending on the duration of your pregnancy, your doctor will guide you towards a medical or surgical method for an MTP.

Note: By law in India, as per the Medical Termination of Pregnancy (Amendment) Bill 2020, an MTP is permissible up to 20 weeks and extended up to 24 weeks of pregnancy if two gynaecologists opine that: (a) there is a possible risk to the physical/mental condition of the mother (this clause includes pregnancy resulting from rape or contraceptive failure); (b) there is a risk of substantial foetal abnormalities.

Some other conditions of concern in pregnancy include **cervical incompetence**, also called cervical insufficiency. It basically means your cervix is dilating (opening up) too early. It increases the risk of a premature birth or leads to pregnancy loss. Earlier than the 28-week mark, preterm labour and delivery is considered very high risk. It is uncommon and occurs only in about 1 per cent of pregnancies. Besides cervical incompetence, preterm premature rupture of the membranes or **PPROM** can also lead to a premature delivery. Simply explained, PPROM is when the amniotic membrane sac breaks earlier than week 37. The signs? A gush or a leak of fluid or even a feeling of wetness in your vagina. PPROM increases your risk of catching infection, which means your doctor will run tests, medicate you and monitor you closely (likely with hospitalization).

Apart from this, pregnancy-induced hypertension that can escalate into pre-eclampsia and also gestational diabetes are among the most common complications in Indian pregnancies. Let's look at these issues in some detail.

Pregnancy-induced hypertension (PIH)

PIH is also called gestational hypertension. It is high BP that is caused because of pregnancy – any time post 20 weeks. Here, your BP reading will be higher than 140/90. But one high BP reading doesn't mean you have hypertension. Your BP must be high on more than two occasions six hours apart when you are resting. And you will not have proteinuria (excess protein in the urine).

How do you get PIH? (1) For no reason, on its own; (2) if you have had high BP pre-pregnancy; (3) you have a kidney disease, immune disorder or diabetes; (4) a previous pregnancy with PIH; (5) you're an older mom; (6) you're carrying multiple babies.

How do you know you have PIH? (1) Sudden weight gain and oedema; (2) you're urinating small amounts; (3) increased BP reading; (4) blurred vision, nausea or vomiting.

Is it harmful? No, if you keep it under check with proper

nutrition (low sodium diet), physical activity and your doctor's advice with regular monitoring and BP medicines. It usually recedes post birth, 12 or so weeks after delivery. Your doctor may choose to deliver your baby early if you have PIH.

When does it become risky? When PIH turns into a severe form of eclampsia, which – among other things – can even cause seizures. Unchecked PIH can affect your placenta and the nutrient supply to your baby. It can also cause a kidney, liver or blood clotting issue.

It is important to bear in mind that 10 to 25 per cent women globally progress from PIH to pre-eclampsia, which is a dangerous condition.

How is PIH different from pre-eclampsia?

Pre-eclampsia is when you have PIH with proteins in your urine – i.e., more than 300 mg recorded in one day. It is basically a sudden upward spike in your BP – above 140/90 – recorded at least twice with a minimum four-hour gap in between. You may feel a pain in the upper right part of your abdomen or severe headaches. The other manifestations and risks in pre-eclampsia are pretty much the same as in PIH. Your doctor may advise additional blood work and choose to deliver your baby earlier.

Gestational diabetes

Also known as Gestational Diabetes Mellitus (GDM), it is a form of high blood sugar that affects pregnant women. The hormones from your placenta basically block your insulin, which is the key in regulating your body's metabolism and sugars. GDM has no major physical symptoms other than excess urination, excess thirst and fatigue. Your OGTT (Oral Glucose

Tolerance Test) blood test of trimester two is usually indicative of gestational diabetes, which means it can be diagnosed post 24 to 28 weeks of pregnancy. A 2017 study indicated that GDM stands at 26.3 per cent in India, which makes Indian women pretty susceptible.

How do you get GDM? Here is a quick list: (1) diabetic pre-pregnancy; (2) older mom; (3) pregnant with multiple babies; (4) overweight; (5) high level of abdominal fat; (6) inactive pregnancy; (7) bed rest during pregnancy.

The risks of GDM? For the mom: (1) type 2 diabetes and/or cardiac issues later in life; (2) obesity; (3) recurrent infections; (4) low blood sugar (hypoglycemia) or very high sugar causing ketosis and coma.

How do you keep it in check? Follow your doctor's advice to the T. Good nutrition, regular physical activity, blood sugar monitoring and blood sugar medication are key.

ANAEMIA: IT's A LOT MORE COMMON THAN YOU'D THINK

What is anaemia? It is a condition in which a person has an insufficient number of red blood cells or reduced haemoglobin. Iron deficiency anaemia is the most common form of anaemia in Indian women. During pregnancy, it is pretty normal for women to develop mild anaemia. However, for some women, a significant iron or B12 or folate deficiency too may cause severe anaemia. During pregnancy, you need more iron and folic acid than usual. Why is that? (1) You use iron to make haemoglobin (i.e., blood) for your baby and yourself and to transfer oxygen across your body. (2) You use folic acid for placental cell growth, and it is an important element in preventing anaemia.

What happens in anaemia? Lower counts of red blood cells essentially reduce the capacity of the blood to carry oxygen. Some of the symptoms of anaemia are fatigue, weakness, dizziness, pale skin, poor immunity, shortness of breath and/or cold hands and feet.

What can you do? An inadequate intake of iron, folic acid and also vitamins B9 and B12 is the most frequent cause. For pregnant and lactating women, 27–45 mg of iron and 400–600 mcg of folic acid are required interventions. There are a few tips that every doctor, expert and nutritionist will give you: (1) Consume iron-rich foods, (2) have vitamin B12 and folic acid supplements, (3) reduce tea and coffee (especially post meals as it reduces the absorption of iron from foods), (4) up your dose of vitamin C to improve iron absorption (see box 'How do I optimize the absorption of all my vitamins?' in Chapter 1: Your First Trimester).

India has had an anaemia control programme since 1970, yet India's National Family Health Survey (NFHS) found that some 50.4 per cent of pregnant women were anaemic in a 2016 survey. About 20 per cent of maternal deaths are a result of anaemia. To diagnose anaemia, your doctor will ask you to get some blood tests and also a physical examination. The blood tests are simple: CBC (complete blood count) and red blood cell morphology. During and post delivery, excessive blood loss can also cause anaemia.

Preparations for trimester two

Birth process

There is no hard-and-fast rule when it comes to preparing for birth. If there is a good prenatal class available to you locally – which suits your budget and sensibility – you could consider joining it. This is where you can go over specifics on labour, breastfeeding and prenatal exercises. However, you will also be able to tap into a wide array of resources online. If you're considering birthing with the assistance of a doula or hypnobirth practitioner or even a water birth, now is the right time to line up all your names. But remember, while these are increasingly fashionable options, they are still not prevalent everywhere in India. Look up hypnobirthing assistants or water birth centres in the city where you live (see section 'Alternate birthing' in Part II: Labour and Childbirth, and What Comes Immediately After). Speak to your ob-gyn for a doula-assisted birth, if you are interested in seeking the services of a doula.

WHAT IS A BIRTHING PLAN? DO I NEED ONE?

A birth plan is entirely optional! It is a lot more common in the West and is only very slowly becoming fashionable in some big Indian cities. Now what does this birthing plan entail? It is a little dossier that communicates pretty much everything you want from your childbirth experience: for example, whether you want an epidural/pain medication or not; what your goals are for labour and childbirth. In a vaginal birth, do you want an episiotomy (where your doctor cuts you) or would you prefer nature to take its course. What is the role of a partner and the assistance of a doula? Some women may have stipulations on placenta removal or about the use of an IV during childbirth, and so on. It is good to bear in mind that in India any birthing plan you will submit to your ob-gyn will come with the caveat that your doctor will make the final decision for you. He/She will try and respect your birthing plan, but if there is a risk or a snap decision involved, your doctor knows best.

Is there a shopping list?

I had a really fun run of stylish clothes when I was pregnant with Taimur. But in Jeh's time, the minute I started getting bigger, I happily swapped to larger-sized underwear, I packed up my jeans and grabbed a series of kaftans that I lived in during my pregnancy and after.

For you: Sure you can update your wardrobe if you need to. But you don't need to go running for maternity clothes. Even larger-sized clothes from normal stores will work for you. And in fact many moms manage their pregnancy wearing their clothes that still fit them – those comfy sweatpants and that worn-out salwar kameez will still be your best friend if you want it to be. There isn't any need for additional shopping unless you really require it (see Chapter 10: Self-Care).

If your belly is growing rapidly, try drawstring or elasticized waists. A lot of you may need to reach for pants with belly bands if you're exercising very regularly – for that bit of extra support. You may already be feeling itchy or hot and will also find that you are naturally drawn towards clothes that feel really comfortable on your skin. Many moms find they need to buy some new lingerie at this point – it is absolutely normal for you to go up a size.

This is a good time to pick up a nice pregnancy pillow (or two) to help you sleep better. You will need more specific products for yourself and your baby towards the end of your pregnancy (see Part III: Getting Ready for the Baby: Your Definitive Guide to Shopping and Planning for the Nursery).

For baby: Now is not the time to rush into any baby shopping. It's still early. What you could do is start making your preliminary list. In fact, it may be a good idea to have your list ready before a baby shower (in case you are planning one) because a bunch of friends and family will want to gift you things you may need. If you are going to have a special nursery, now is the time to start modelling it. You can start shopping some time in trimester three, depending on how anxious you feel about being prepared.

WHAT'S THE BIG FUSS ABOUT A PREGNANCY PILLOW?

I wouldn't have lasted a minute without this pregnancy sleeping pillow of mine. I would take a selfie with it if I could! Towards the end of term, sleeping was like death. I am usually a back sleeper, and staying on my side through the night was a challenge. The pillow was crucial to my sanity.

Forget about husbands, most pregnant women save all their devotion and hugs for their pregnancy pillows during this time! And why not? Sleep becomes harder as your bump grows, and a body pillow becomes necessary for side sleeping with comfort. The idea is to nest yourself, curl into and wrap your legs around a large (three to four foot) U-shaped or C-shaped pillow. There is a world of options available on Amazon India and other online marketplaces like Flipkart, which is likely your easiest choice. Alternatively, many mums have happily walked into their nearest bedding store and ordered customized pillows for themselves.

Another option is a four- to five-foot long straight pillow which is useful to simply wrap your legs around so that you can orient yourself to the side while sleeping. Use a regular pillow to wedge under your lower back in this case, so you are not scared about rolling on to your back while you sleep.

A sloped 'wedge' pillow can also be helpful for back support: (a) while you sit, (b) to place under your growing belly as you sleep, and (c) to put your head on (slightly elevated) to help with acid reflux when you're lying down.

Can I sleep on my stomach?

You can sleep on your stomach easily during your first trimester. You will not be putting pressure on your baby. But as you move on to the second and third trimesters and your bump begins to grow, it may actually be physically inconvenient to do so. Issues like indigestion and heartburn and, later, pressure on the vena cava (i.e., the main vein that pumps blood from your heart to your legs) will make sleeping on your stomach practically impossible. So, don't worry about accidentally sleeping on your tummy. You won't!

Music? Chants? What is pregnancy listening?

I did not listen to any chants, prayers or meditations when I was pregnant. But I did listen to a lot of jazz! From Nat King Cole and Louis Armstrong to Aretha Franklin and Nina Simone. This is the music, the 'listening' that transports me to a different world. That, for me, is therapeutic. It's meditation! I think every woman just needs to figure out what brings her peace and follow that. It doesn't have to be a mantra or a chant! Even a favourite rock album can calm you down.

Post 21 weeks is a good time to get started on exposing your abdomen to meditative/religious chants, prayers, classical music or even just good old rock 'n' roll, if that's your vibe. Strap a good pair of headphones directly on to your abdomen while you continue your day's work, chores or meditation! This is when your baby is able to catch sounds.

Music, spiritual chants and guided meditations can have a calming effect, thereby lowering your stress levels and easing anxiety. The more relaxed you are, the better it is for your baby. As your baby begins to hear the sounds around you, she will also begin to respond to them. So why not create a soothing, happy pregnancy playlist for both of you?

You will find a host of pregnancy listening lists online, including those tailored for different religions and communities. For example, Garbh Sanskar (a Sanskrit term for 'education in the womb') chants are popular with Hindu families.

Finances

Get the niggling things out of the way right now. Like post-baby budget planning with your partner. Recee your hospital expenses. Check what your medical insurance covers. Get your bank account in place.

How do I figure things out at work?

If your pregnancy is going well, you can work till the day before you deliver your baby. Just do simple things to make your day more comfortable. Take frequent breaks to walk around. Dress easy, eat healthy and drink a lot of water. Arrange for a small pouf or footstool so you can put up your feet. Discuss your pregnancy with your employer/employees and colleagues. If too much is being demanded of you, learn to say no. If you are planning to take a complete break from work post baby, now is the time to inform the people you work with. Figure out your maternity leave options at this stage.

Note: As per the Maternity Benefit (Amendment) Act, 2017, your company should inform you in writing about the maternity benefits available to you at the time you join them. Most workplaces have to offer maternity benefits unless it is a company with ten or less employees. You have a right to a 26-week maternity leave. This can be taken towards the end of your pregnancy or can begin post delivery. By law, if the nature of your work is appropriate, you should be allowed to work from home in addition to the maternity benefit period. If you have completed a minimum of 80 days at work in the 12 months preceding your delivery, your maternity leave is awarded with full pay. You cannot be dismissed for taking maternity leave. In case you are dismissed, your company is liable to pay you for medical and maternity expenses.

End of trimester two: Quick look

Baby: Your baby is 14 inches long, weighs up to 0.9 kg and is a fully formed little baby with an active sense of taste and hearing. Her eyes are blinking, she is kicking up her feet and grabbing with her fist. All the organs are fully developed, including a brain that is fully functional.

Mom: Your uterus has grown upwards and outwards, and you have a pronounced baby bump. On an average, you would have gained 0.2 to 0.5 kg a week (or approximately 0.75 kg per week, with multiple babies). This was the most easy-going phase of your pregnancy – in terms of how you felt. If you started out your pregnancy in a normal weight range, you are likely to be 5 to 7 kg up. A maximum of 9 kg is acceptable if you started off skinny; and 5 to 6 kg if you were overweight before you got pregnant.

3

YOUR THIRD TRIMESTER

I think I had only one fear during my first pregnancy: the prospect of breastfeeding! I was paranoid. Would I get enough milk? Would my baby latch? I don't know why it scared me so much. But I know that breastfeeding is a common anxiety for a lot of first-time mums. It was my doctor who told me to relax. He said we will cross the bridge when we get there, that we will make sure it happens. And you know the best part? He reassured me that even if doesn't happen – it's okay. What did I learn at the end of trimester three? Well, two boys, two pregnancies, two different experiences, two very different babies and two different moms too! That was it, in a nutshell.

You're in the final stretch of your pregnancy now, inching closer to the finish line. Most of you will find yourself tiring faster. You are also going to be feeling excited and anxious, and might find yourself tossing and turning at night with all kinds of thoughts. You will soon be meeting your baby, after all – the heart of all the anticipation that's been building up since week one!

The **third trimester of your pregnancy** is from week 29 to week 40 – which is months seven, eight and nine. If you are beginning to get nervous about labour, take heart that you're not alone. Most women fear the process of birthing and worry about it as D-Day gets closer; in fact, for most women, it's the single biggest worry.

Many of the symptoms we flagged in trimester two might show up at this point. It is very common to feel fatigue or shortness of breath and have trouble sleeping during this phase. These symptoms all work on each other and occur in a sort of vicious cycle, just like haemorrhoids and constipation – another unpleasant pair. Urinary incontinence, mood swings, leaky breasts and heartburn are also very common. Most women feel their first hints of Braxton-Hicks contractions during trimester three. But there is no fixed rule regarding this. You may not even feel a single contraction-like movement until you are actually in labour.

This is the trimester where your body will really change as your bump grows fast and your weight gain increases. This isn't always an uphill ratio though; many women find that their weight plateaus during the end of trimester three. Your little one is also raring to go. You will really feel his movements and you'll start counting his kicks. You might be tempted to pore over your ultrasound to figure out if you're having a boy or a girl. Mostly everyone tries! Just remember you probably won't be able to decipher your ultrasound! If you're a second-time mum, the beginning of trimester three is a great time to start explaining the new addition to your firstborn (see section 'Preparations for trimester three').

You will most likely be delivering your baby at a hospital or at a nursing home. Based on the norms that the hospital/nursing home follows, you may have already registered in advance for the birth of your baby. If you haven't done it so far, your seventh month is when you will be asked to register yourself and pay for the room. Your doctor will guide you in the registration process (see box 'Registering for your delivery' in Chapter 1: Your First Trimester).

What's of primary importance in trimester three? The first is your baby's position and the measurement parameters in your ultrasounds, as this ascertains the outcome of childbirth or, at the least, provides a clearer picture of where you're headed.

The second is your baby's movements. Moms are encouraged to be attentive and attuned to their baby's movements on a daily basis (see box 'Do you need to be counting your baby's kicks?'). Women with high-risk pregnancies are told to keep a count of the kicks and inform the doctor if they feel less than 10 movements in a day.

The third is developing an awareness about signs of labour as the big day arrives. The earliest signs of labour can kick in a few weeks or a few hours before actual childbirth (see Chapter 4: Labour and Childbirth).

This is the trimester to read up on labour, watch videos or join a prenatal or birthing class (if one is available to you locally) to prepare for childbirth and childcare. It's also a great time to start tackling your shopping lists, practise Lamaze, prepare your hospital bag (towards the end) and finish any house-related work.

PRETERM, FULL TERM, POST TERM: WHAT DO ALL THESE VARIOUS WEEKS MEAN?

We have already read about premature births in the trimester two section of this book. It might help to keep a few more of these numbers in mind as we enter trimester three. Studies have shown that pregnancy can naturally vary by up to five weeks from person to person.

- If you're carrying twins, you are likely to deliver at 35 to 36 weeks – it is normal and healthy; 37 weeks is considered 'full term' for twins, on average.
- In case you're carrying triplets, your average pregnancy length will be about 32 weeks.
- If you are carrying a single baby, your baby will no longer be categorized as 'preterm' from 37 completed weeks. Officially, a 'full-term' single baby is one that is born anywhere between 37–40 weeks. And 41–42 weeks and beyond is called a 'late-term' or 'post-term' baby.
- For a single baby, labour and childbirth at the 38-week-stage (give or take a few days) is extremely common on a global average.
- A very small percentage of women deliver after the 'whole nine months' (40 weeks).
- Most women do not deliver on their exact EDD either – a 10-day variable period is common.

A look at the third trimester for an IVF mom

As we discussed across trimesters one and two, an IVF mom has medical protocols similar to those of a natural pregnancy. What differs is that you may continue to have one additional routine ultrasound per trimester and definitely a couple of extra ultrasounds if you are carrying multiple babies. Remember that a pregnancy achieved through any assisted reproductive technology is not considered high risk. But you may be placed under stricter care if you're an older mom, have a complicated reproductive history, have a precious pregnancy or are carrying multiple babies. This is completely normal. In case you are pregnant with multiple babies, your doctor will continue to keep a close eye on your cervical measurements. Be prepared to deliver your twins earlier than what is considered 'full term' for singleton babies.

What's happening to your body in the third trimester?

There were so many nights when I just couldn't sleep – I was anxious, excited, nervous and scared. It happens to all of us! I felt this from my eighth month during both my pregnancies. My sleep patterns were so haywire that I was tired during the day. My energy would slump from 5 p.m. I would get into bed by a very respectable 11 p.m., but I would be tossing and turning till 3 a.m. I had at least three nightly loo runs and I'd be up but groggy from 7 a.m. I think I survived my last two months on nothing more than random snoozes through the day.

This is the trimester when you will suddenly look and feel much bigger. Starting from day 0 and going up until the very end of your pregnancy, your uterus expands to between 20 and 30 times its normal size. Did you know it goes from weighing 35–50 grams pre-pregnancy to becoming round, hard and a little over 1 kg at the time you give birth? At the end of term (on an average), not only is your blood volume high, but your placenta weighs in at 0.7 kg, the amniotic fluid adds up to 0.8 kg (roughly half a litre), your breast tissue would be about 0.9 to 1.3 kg, the stored fat (for delivery and breastfeeding) may go from 2.2 to 4 kg and your baby could weigh from 2.5 kg up to 4 kg.

As you ease into week 29, many of your organs – stomach and diaphragm mainly – will start getting squeezed by your expanding uterus. It's a major smush-and-squeeze show for your organs actually, right from trimester one when your bladder first gets squished. In trimester three, your liver and lungs (which used to be lower in your torso) are getting squeezed by your stomach and intestines. Slower digestion, breathlessness and heartburn are just some of the side effects of this, which you might have begun to see in the second trimester.

From weeks 31 to 33, the amniotic fluid in your uterus is at its maximum. It will then start reducing gradually post 35 weeks. By now your placenta is pretty much an organ in its own right, as it grows steadily with your baby through the nine months. Your labour is technically only over once you deliver the placenta after delivering your baby.

From week 34 or so, your weight gain might start slowing down. It's perfectly fine. You don't need to up your eating. All pregnant women do not gain weight at a consistent rate.

Post the 36-week mark, your baby may drop lower into your pelvis and ease the pressure you felt so far on your lungs. This is called 'lightening' or 'baby dropping'. It is when the widest part of your baby's head shifts lower into your pelvis in preparation for birth – and gets 'engaged' (see box 'What does "engaging" mean?'). It is not an indication of when your labour process will begin. For many women, this happens two to four weeks before labour, and for many it happens at the time of labour. You will see a visible downward shift in your bump and you will feel more pressure on your rectum and pelvic floor. While the pressure on your lungs will ease and you might get less heartburn, it may kick up your bathroom rounds and urinary incontinence.

This is also the time your amniotic fluid will begin to decrease gradually. By 42 weeks, it is too low – though chances are your baby has come out a while before that! Worried that your baby is still in a breech position? By week 37, most babies will have turned, and moved head down to the correct position. If, however, your baby remains in breech at week 38, you will have to put yourself down for an elective Caesarean.

Trimester three sees a flux of hormones, all working solo or in tandem with each other to help you reach the end of term. At around the 32-week mark, your body's oestrogen and progesterone levels peak to the highest ever for trimester three. So, what changes can you expect? Ankle swellings and mood swings, to name a few. Relaxin is still at play – which means your ligaments are loosening, and joint aches are common.

Let's now meet some other hormones. The hormone that helps you make breast milk is called prolactin and it amps up towards the end of trimester three and especially postpartum – going up to 10 times in level. If your breasts leak during trimester three, you are secreting colostrum. This is the start of your breast milk. It is a little yellowish in colour and it is what you will first be feeding your baby when you begin nursing. The trimester three leak happens when your prolactin levels outrun your oestrogen and progesterone.

Then, as you inch towards the big day, your oxytocin rises while progesterone drops. Oxytocin is the hormone that causes increased contractions of the uterus and stimulates milk into the breast ducts. Oxytocin plays its most important role during labour, particularly in pushing the placenta out post childbirth and helping stave off excess bleeding.

In case your labour needs to be induced, your doctor will give you a dose of synthetic oxytocin (called pitocin). It is this oxytocin that works with oestrogen towards softening your cervix to prepare for childbirth too (see Chapter 4: Labour and Childbirth to understand more about inducing labour).

As you reach the end of term, your cervix will start softening. If you haven't already felt any Braxton-Hicks contractions yet, you may just start now. If Braxton-Hicks contractions do not make any appearance through your pregnancy – that is also fine. You may lose your mucus plug towards the end of your term. If you lose it much earlier, it may indicate that you're going into preterm labour. For some women, the mucus plug expels just before their water breaks (see section 'A glossary of labour terms' in Chapter 4: Labour and Childbirth).

Remember, if you develop abdominal cramps, severe back pain, dizziness or bleeding – you have to call your doctor right away.

WHAT DOES 'ENGAGING' MEAN?

We've already discussed the occipito-anterior position of the baby – i.e., the ideal position for birthing. Your baby can get into this position without actually 'engaging'. Foetal head engagement is a specific term used by the ob-gyn to denote the largest diameter of the foetal head entering the maternal pelvic outlet. It also serves as a reassurance to the doctors that the foetal head size is not too big for the passage it is supposed to go through and that a vaginal delivery is a distinct possibility. There are different points of time at which foetal head engagement happens. It is two weeks earlier for first-time moms; and most often during delivery for second- or third-time moms. Head engagement

> means there is a good chance of vaginal delivery because it rules out a condition called cephalopelvic disproportion or CPD (where the foetal head is bigger than the maternal pelvis and requires a Caesarean delivery).

What's your baby up to?

It is those end-of-term ultrasounds that are the real deal. I'm so glad I did every test by the book, otherwise I think I would have headed into an emergency situation. With Taimur, we caught the nuchal cords (looped around his neck) at the right time and hurriedly opted for a Caesarean. With Jeh, I knew I would most likely end up on the Caesarean table because I had had one before, but it wasn't until I was a proper 40 weeks in. He was very high, even at 40 weeks. Had I even wanted to wait for labour to occur naturally, it wouldn't have.

A QUICK END-OF-MONTH SUMMARY

Month 7
Key milestone? Fat development; functional organs; eyes that open and close
What's the average size? 14 inches
What's the average weight? Approximately 0.9–1.8 kg

Month 8
Key milestone? Lungs are fully developed by the end; bones are strengthened; quick weight gain

What's the average size? 18 inches
What's the average weight? Up to 2.27 kg

Month 9
Key milestone? All reflexes are coordinated
What's the average size? 18–20 inches
What's the average weight? Up to 4 kg

Week 29: Your baby is about 33 cm long. He can open his eyes and can 'focus', which means he is prepping for the eye contact he's going to make with you soon. His body is getting less and less wrinkly as fat develops under the skin. Your baby is sleeping 90 to 95 per cent of the time in your womb. But not all these hours are spent in deep sleep though. Your baby can move in his sleep too, so you can expect to feel movement.

Week 30: You remember the vernix and lanugo on your baby's skin that showed up in trimester two? That will slowly begin to disappear. Those little kidneys are now completely functional, which means your baby's pee is regularly flowing into the amniotic fluid. His lungs continue to develop through this phase. He is prepping for that first gasp of breath, that first cry which is going to happen shortly. Your baby has kissable cheeks already!

Week 31: This is the stage from where you and your doctor will start paying attention to the baby's movements (see box 'Do you need to be counting your baby's kicks?'). There is no set pattern of movement – your baby's not always going to be resting when you are! On an average, your baby should likely be putting on

200 grams per week from now. Your little one's soft cartilage is strengthening into bone – he's getting stronger!

Week 32: Those fingernails are getting longer, and your baby is going to need his first trim pretty soon post birth! It is said that your baby is a lot more sensitive to sound by now – which explains why babies can respond to the sounds of their mothers' voices from birth. For a lot of mums, the baby gets into the occipito-anterior (ideal for natural birth) position by now, i.e., they have their head down, their face looking to your back, chin tucked in and legs up.

Week 33: That former see-through X-Men-like skin is slowly becoming opaque. Did you know that your baby's skull is soft and pliant at this stage, so it can assist in his descent through the birth canal? The skull protects the brain by moving and readjusting during the birthing process so that your baby can make his way through easily. What's more, the nervous system is now completely up and running.

Week 34: If you caught a glimpse of your baby now, he looks as snug as a bug – feet curled up, knees to chest. Your breech baby can turn laterally or fully during these last few weeks. He's quite a flexible little gymnast now! By this time, this little thing is already producing the enzymes that will help process food within his digestive tract post birth.

Week 35: Feel a sudden ease in the pressure on your lungs? Your baby might drop down into your pelvis in preparation for birth any time from this week on. It's called 'lightening'. The little one is also continually building his own storehouse of fat. This is what is going to help him regulate his body temperature when out in the world. Do you know your baby is no longer fully visible in an ultrasound image? Your sonologist will be rolling the transducer across your abdomen to check different parts of your baby one at a time.

Week 36: If your baby is born any time **after** this phase, he may not even need external help with breathing in the beginning (like preterm babies generally would). Your baby's lungs are now fully developed and in a deflated position and are deriving oxygen from your placenta. Those little lungs will inflate at his first gasp of air. His heart is beating at 110 to 160 beats per minute – this is normal in vitro. Do you know this won't change post birth? In fact, your baby's heart rate remains at 80 to 140 beats per minute till the age of five. (P.S.: The normal adult heart rate is 60 to 100 beats per minute.)

Week 37: A baby born at the completion of a full 37 weeks is considered 'full term' (i.e., even '36 weeks and 4 days' is considered 'preterm'). Twins born three to four weeks early are a fairly common occurrence. It is rare that a preterm twin baby doesn't end up in the NICU, however. It's fine. Your doctor will tell you in advance to stay prepared for a stay in the NICU.

Week 38: In case you have twins and still haven't gone into labour, you may be induced for birth to minimize health risks to your babies. During this week, your little one will be gaining more fat. His lanugo will now disappear. The vernix remains to assist his descent through the birth canal during a vaginal delivery. By this stage, your little one is taking every chance he gets to practise suckling – thumb, fingers, hands!

Week 39: This little person in your tummy is exactly the same one you will meet. Just because space is getting tight, it doesn't mean your baby is uncomfortable or cannot move. You will feel his movements till the very end. Your baby can show up any time till week 40 or 42. It's just a waiting game.

Week 40: For a few weeks now, your baby has developed coordination with his reflexes. That means he can already do a lot of the stuff he's meant to do when out in the real world: grasp, blink, turn his head, respond to sound and light. Yes, it starts this early!

Do you need to be counting your baby's kicks?

In the earlier stages of your pregnancy, you don't feel your baby move that much. The flutters and quickening are sporadic, gentle and difficult to keep track of (see box 'Flutters or quickening' from Chapter 2: Your Second Trimester). However, post the sixth and seventh month of pregnancy, your baby's movements are more pronounced, and it is important to watch out for these.

Why? If there is a sudden increase in foetal movement – like a flurry of activity – sustained for a couple hours or so, it could be a sign that your baby is in distress. On the other hand, if there are no movements at all for an extended period of time – like, say, 24 hours or more – it could be another cause for worry. In both cases, you need to speak to your doctor.

Counting kicks gained a lot of momentum from 2008, with a stillbirth prevention public health campaign (in the

US), called 'Count the Kicks'. It was inspired from public health research conducted in Norway, which showed that teaching pregnant moms to monitor foetal movement in trimester three reduced the risk of stillbirth by 30 per cent.

Now, when people talk about a baby's kicks, it doesn't mean a strong 'kick in the gut' kind of kick for everyone. Many moms feel only mild movements till the very end. Your baby's kicks, jabs, swishes, turns, rolls and pokes are in totality an indication that all is well, or a potential red flag of foetal distress.

So, how do you do this?

1. If you read up on the 'Count the Kicks' protocol, the advice is to note down the number of minutes it took you to count approximately 10 movements. Sit comfortably with your feet up or lie down on your side (the left side is best). It is okay if it takes up to two hours to record 10 movements. Pick another time later that day to try this exercise if it doesn't work the first time. Try the do-over post another snack or activity spell. This is definitely one solid way of doing it. However, if you ask your doctor (or paediatrician) locally, they are likelier to tell you that there is no fixed number of movements – each baby is different. Rather than literally 'counting' movements, be mindful of your baby's usual movements every day. The baby sleeps for over 20 hours a day, so don't start worrying if there is no movement in, say, two or three hours.

2. Maintain a chart on your own or look up a 'kick count chart' online and use it.

3. Pick the approximate same time every day for this activity, when you have noticed a pattern of movement in your baby. Do this after a snack, meal or some physical activity. Many doctors do not recommend that low-risk pregnant women count their kicks daily as it causes unnecessary worry.

4. Moms who have an anterior placenta position (i.e., placenta is near the stomach), or who are overweight, may have some difficulty in charting their baby's movements.

5. As your pregnancy advances and your baby has limited space to move around, these movements may become less pronounced. But the movements will still be there.

How will I feel: Symptoms of trimester three

My Braxton-Hicks contractions showed up midway through trimester three during both my pregnancies. I could also feel the baby's head turn. Sleeping was like death! I would be awake half the night, anxious that I would roll over on to my back in my sleep!

Let's recollect everything we talked about earlier in trimesters one and two – right from heartburn, round ligament pain, ankle swellings and stretch marks to frequent urination, numb hands, sweating and haemorrhoids. You can expect any, all or some of these symptoms to show up in trimester three. Oh, and did we mention this includes bleeding gums, extreme heat, headaches and light-headedness too? Braxton-Hicks contractions and

SPD – check. Leaky breasts and darkening skin patches – also check. Lower back pain, breathlessness and sleepless nights – big checks.

Your shifting centre of gravity has begun to weigh down on your abdominal muscles, giving you bad back pain. If you have spent a lot of your pregnancy on bed rest, you may have an especially tough run of things with your back.

Those round ligament pains act up at night with the odd leg cramp. You may have swelling, due to oedema. It's a combination of the weight you're carrying, your crazy hormones, the things you're thinking (and stressing) about, and the sleepless nights as you try and find a comfortable angle for your body.

You are already feeling some amount of fatigue by the time you reach trimester three – and these three months are quite likely to escalate those feelings. Many of these correlate, actually, as the pain and swelling keep you up at night and the insomnia tires you by day.

The pressure on your lungs can make you feel breathless, and this feeling of trying to catch your breath actually adds to the exhaustion. The acid reflux and heartburn aren't doing much to help you relax either. All these factors that were discussed across trimesters one and two come into heightened play now.

Remember, your heart is also working harder than normal – your heart rate increases by 10 to 20 beats per minute during pregnancy. This can cause you to feel palpitations, dizziness, shortness of breath and, again, exhaustion. What can you do? Just try and get as much rest as you can. And tell yourself this is your last leg!

If you fall in the tiny category of mums who feel none of this except some exhaustion and trouble with sleeping positions, you're definitely privileged. But if you're not, don't feel cheated. It's just par for the course!

False labour aka Braxton-Hicks contractions

You'll hear this term over and over again, so let's take a look at what it is. These contractions are called prodromal or 'false labour' pains. They can make their first appearance in trimester two (especially in second and third pregnancies). However, they are much more common in trimester three. Again, like all symptoms, not all women experience them.

What happens during a Braxton-Hicks contraction? You will feel a tightening of the muscles across your belly. It is your body preparing (or, you can say, rehearsing) for true labour. It does not mean that labour has started. If you touch your stomach during a Braxton-Hicks contraction, you will feel like it is hard because the muscles of your uterus are contracting and tightening. These contractions are basically irregular and random and don't increase in intensity or occur closer together (in terms of time) the way 'true labour' contractions do. Braxton-Hicks contractions are not associated with pain.

Each contraction may last about 30 to 60 seconds (or for a maximum of two minutes). The contractions could go on for a few hours or end very quickly. They may crop up in trimester two and linger, or start in trimester three and stay till the end. They don't have a pattern/schedule. While they occur spontaneously, here are some triggers that pregnant women have noted: (a) dehydration, (b) full bladder, (c) sexual activity, (d) increase in physical activity and also (e) an increase in baby movements.

What can you do to ease things? Change your activity: rest if you have been on your feet, or take a walk if you have been lying down. Drink water and get a snack. Try mildly warm packs, water bags or a bath. Try and do a few breathing exercises to relax your body.

Note: If you feel like you have passed fluids or have an accompanying back pain or feel like you want to pass stool, call your doctor.

How do you differentiate between Braxton-Hicks and true labour?

Timing is everything! True labour contractions that indicate impending childbirth: (a) become stronger in intensity (i.e., pain), (b) happen at intervals that can be timed, (c) start to happen at closer intervals as labour progresses, (d) occur in waves. While labour pains aren't expected till 37 weeks, if they do start early (preterm), there are some other signs that your body is going into true labour: (1) your 'water breaks' – meaning you begin to leak amniotic fluid in a trickle or a sudden gush, (2) you pass your cervical mucus plug – it could be a stringy or sticky mucus-like discharge and clear, pinkish or blood-tinged in colour.

How will I look?

I watched my body change drastically and I didn't care. I am not a small built or skinny girl! There are so many moms who hardly gain any weight at all except on their belly. But my body is different. I ballooned during both pregnancies. Even my hands and feet grew in my last trimester! But I didn't feel embarrassed about it. I wore fitted gym clothes and shot for Puma during my eighth month in Jeh's time.

And I refused to allow them to airbrush anything or choose flattering angles. So what if I looked fat?

You mean apart from all the pleasant and not-so-fun manifestations of pregnancy you read about in trimesters one and two? Like everything from curves and lush hair to stretch marks, swollen ankles, linea nigra and darkening skin patches? No, it's all covered!

Your belly will be big! At some point of time in your pregnancy, it may even feel like it is growing a little bit every day. People will tell you you're carrying high, low or wide; that your belly is small, big, round or pointy. Does that mean anything? Basically, no. It has no implications for the weight, size or gender of your baby. Some moms find their bumps are smaller in their first pregnancies compared to their second. Additionally, sometimes shorter moms find their bumps protrude outwards more than taller moms – perhaps because their torsos are shorter.

Globally, **11 to 15 kg of weight gain by the end of trimester three** is common and acceptable. If you started your pregnancy underweight or overweight or if you're carrying multiple babies, your parameters will definitely differ. These days, **a trendy global norm is 9 to 11 kg of total weight gain** at the end of pregnancy. Please note this is not always achievable! A maximum 0.45 kg weekly weight gain is fine. If you have any underlying health complications or, again, for overweight mums, your doctor will keep a close check on weight gain anyway.

It is also normal for weight gain to slow down in the last trimester. A lot of women do not gain much weight in their last month. Some even end up shedding a kilo or two. Also, you won't gain weight evenly. The bulk of your weight will quite likely be on your back, hips and upper thighs. There are no golden rules here. Enjoy these last three months. This is how things are, and this is how you look!

Your emotions

Your hormones continue to shift and churn. Your body is changing so rapidly. There is a lot on your mind, and your life is about to change. It is absolutely fine to feel overwhelmed. It is also absolutely fine to not be able to name your feelings or talk about them clearly. Is it excitement or anxiety? Stress or fear? A little bit of everything perhaps?

Trimester three is when you should really start planning for your baby in terms of his needs within your home. You know when people say 'reality strikes'? This is it! You're going to be a mom! And this feeling, this sense of impending responsibility, can be overwhelming. You'll wonder what sort of parent you'll be. You'll wonder if you're likely to fail. Can you fail? No! Being a mom is something you learn on the job, you land on your feet and keep running. The wonders are all yours, the mistakes you make are also all yours.

Childbirth is the leading cause of fear among most women. There is the fear of handling the pain of a vaginal birth or worries over a Caesarean. You know that feeling of nervousness in the pit of your stomach before a big exam? It may just take you back to those days in school. Writing your thoughts down might relieve some of those anxieties. Make lists – shopping, to-do, exercises, meditation targets and work deadlines; staying task-oriented might actually give your anxieties a good outlet. The most important thing to remember is that this is the world's most natural process, that countless women have been on this journey. You are not alone.

Those 'raging hormones' can also make you feel emotionally wrought. You may catch yourself fighting with your partner, snapping at a colleague or scolding your older child – and regretting it the next day. Remember, you haven't turned into a monster, and that this is a passing phase. Feeling angry and alienated is very much a real thing – no matter what a rosy little bubble people think your pregnancy is.

Try and figure out where this anger is projecting from. For instance, do you feel your partner isn't as involved or attentive as you'd like? Do you think your family isn't pitching in enough? Do you sense an inequality at your workplace? Your emotions can follow any narrative. This is the right time to just find someone you can talk to about these feelings – your partner, a friend, family or even a counsellor. Your partner can step in at this stage – their role is an important component of your 40 weeks (see box 'Five tips for the partner').

FIVE TIPS FOR THE PARTNER

With Sonali Gupta, clinical psychologist

- As a parent-to-be, it's normal to experience anxiety
- Your presence matters: Make a choice to accompany your partner for her check-ups and ultrasounds
- Have conversations about shared responsibilities: Pregnancy is a good time to start practising this
- Talk about your shared values around parenthood: All decisions around money, upbringing, religion, childcare and support are a function of this
- Mindfully carve out time so that you and your partner can enjoy your time together before your baby is born

Many moms also feel a strong nesting instinct in the third trimester as the due date comes closer. It is basically a compulsive need for you to plan, clean, decorate and prepare for your baby. It could manifest as a mad shopping urge or a manic spring-cleaning spree in your house. It's quite likely because you want everything to be perfect for your little one. Just bear in mind that you are also getting big and are tiring faster, so stop to rest and stay clued in with the signs your body is giving you.

Then there are pregnancy dreams! Have they happened to you already? For a lot of women, pregnancy dreams kick in during trimester three. There is no rocket science behind these dreams, so you don't need to overthink them. Essentially, all your hormones and your emotions – whether joy, fear, ambivalence, uncertainty, anxiety, excitement – need an outlet. Experts say these are what pregnancy dreams are all about. What sort of dreams do most women get? A picture of life with a baby. Crazy sex dreams. Frightening childbirth images. Holidays in Kashmir. Being an all-star parent. Being a terrible parent! Everything is fair game.

I AM TOO SCARED TO HAVE SEX, AND IT'S AFFECTING MY RELATIONSHIP

With Sonali Gupta, clinical psychologist

It's very common for your sex drive and libido to be impacted during your pregnancy. Not just that, different women's bodies respond to the need for sexual intimacy in differing ways, and that's very normal too. My advice would be to be open about concerns around intimacy with your gynaecologist. Very often in my practice, I see that most women are not comfortable or they shy away from asking these questions about either an increase in libido or their fears about intimacy and low sex drive. In my experience, often women who have had a miscarriage tend to be fearful of having sex during their pregnancy. Each pregnancy is unique and so also is how the couple experience intimacy during that period.

Consider these pointers:

- Intimacy and sexual pleasure can exist beyond intercourse/penetrative sex. Figure out creative ways to create intimacy. As partners, lying next to each other, caressing and stroking, giving each other a backrub or a gentle massage are some ways of experiencing intimacy.

- In moments when you don't feel like engaging in sexual intimacy, have a conversation with your partner. Talk to them about what you are feeling: whether it's stress, fatigue or lack of sexual drive that's impacting you. Very often when women choose to not articulate the reasons, the partner may experience a sense of personal rejection.

- Look at each other as sexual partners and not just as parents. This is especially pronounced among second-time moms.

- Try and enjoy your pregnancy as a couple. Build shared moments. It's a milestone. We often forget to enjoy the process and the little moments of connection.

When I was pregnant with Taimur, I was younger and more energetic. I felt fitter. I was out and about and – yes – I had my mojo! But I didn't feel particularly sexy when I was pregnant with Jeh. I was quite a wreck for a good part of my first four months. I noticed a drastic shift in my libido. I read up about it, and it's very common. And I was truly grateful for Saif's support during this time. He was always so understanding. Not every woman feels good. Not every woman feels sexy. And to make love, you need to feel beautiful and feel loved. Any partner needs to understand how women feel with their changing hormones and with carrying a whole life inside them. When you're pregnant, sex often does not feel that important. Even though things eased out for me from my fifth month, my second pregnancy was definitely tough.

What am I allowed to do?

There's a flurry of questions and a frenzy of activity as you begin your countdown to the end. Can you bend or lift? Can you drive, exercise or travel? What about work, sex and your baby shopping list? Let's start with the basics – food, fitness, sex, travel, work and shopping – and then move on to other specific pregnancy FAQs.

Do I have to eat a lot?

A lot of you may feel your appetite decrease as you move towards the end of the pregnancy. That's just because your uterus is pressing down on your organs, and you're feeling heavy and breathless and as if you can't digest your food. Your baby is still being fuelled by your energy, however. So, experts advise not to eat significantly less. You don't have to force-feed yourself or 'eat for two' at any stage. But most moms opt for fluids and smaller portions on the days they are feeling far from hungry. Statistically, you will need 450 to 500 extra calories per day in trimester three. And if you have multiple babies, your calorie requirements are pegged at about 300 calories per baby per day. But rather than get caught up in calculating your calorie intake, stick to the healthy habits you have been following since week one. Indulge your cravings when you feel the need to. This is the final stretch!

Should I exercise?

Most women feel better and more energized when they keep up their physical activity in trimester three. It is completely safe to stay fit and active till the day you deliver. But, this trimester, you will need to be cautious and decrease the intensity of your workouts. Lift weights, but use a lighter load. Walk, but don't elevate your heart rate. Avoid jumping exercises. And completely steer clear of anything that may make you fall or impact your belly very hard. Gentle and correctly done squats can open out your pelvis, help the baby engage and assist in the birthing process. Check with your doctor before you commence on those end-of-term squats or duck walks. For instance, if your baby has moved down and you're still far from end of term, you should avoid squats. Kegels, squats, duck walks and butterfly pose are otherwise considered the holy quad of labour and childbirth.

A lot of you may now feel more comfortable sticking to prenatal yoga, walking, swimming and stretches. It's a great time to look up internationally certified prenatal exercises and get started on what you're comfortable doing. It is important to keep up with your Kegels. Exercise helps in easing some of the discomforts of pregnancy and is a great way to keep up your strength so you get back on your feet faster post delivery (see Chapter 9: Fitness).

Can I have sex?

Yes, safely, till the very end of term, as long as you feel like it. Unless you have any underlying medical conditions (requiring pelvic rest) that your doctor will warn you about – there is no problem. In case you're wondering if your now 'woke' and neurologically functioning baby can figure things out, umm, he won't know or feel a thing! Skim back to the pregnancy sex advice shared in trimesters one and two. Nothing much has changed except your growing belly. More blood is flowing to your cervix during trimester three and it is changing in preparation for childbirth, which is why you may notice some spotting after intercourse. But it is important to report any untoward bleeds, mild or major, to your doctor right away.

Can I travel?

Post your second trimester and the 27–28-week phase, most airlines are quite likely to ask you to carry a letter from your doctor clearing you to fly. A lot of women choose not to travel in their third trimester. Once you cross 36–37 weeks, most airlines will not permit you to fly (this restriction starts sooner if you're carrying twins). Is there a safety issue when it comes to travelling? Perhaps not. But, yes, the chance of going into labour or developing any other end-of-term issues while you're on an airplane, on the road or in a different country – away from your comfort zone, your doctor and your support system – is now fairly high. In general, most women don't travel at this point in their pregnancy, and if you choose to do so, be aware you are taking a risk.

Make sure you have sorted out your travel and medical insurance when you travel. Meet your doctor before you travel to discuss your health and safety. Carry your pregnancy file with your latest reports for extra caution – in your hand luggage would be ideal. Follow the same travel precautions as you did in trimesters one and two. Keep your SOS medicines in your handbag, hydrate, and take frequent breaks to walk around the flight cabin. Your chances of developing a blood clot are higher during this phase of your pregnancy, so compression socks may help on flights.

If you're planning a short trip by road or rail, check the quality of toilets and roads along the way. And if you are travelling to any country which needs a specific vaccine, check if it is pregnancy safe or not. This advice, of course, holds true for travel across your pregnancy.

What's my life at work?

If you have a healthy pregnancy, you can literally work till the last day of your pregnancy. You can also happily opt to take the last few weeks off. Many mums choose to work till the day they go to the hospital and use their entire maternity leave post delivery. Find the option that works best for you and your situation. Follow the advice from trimester two – like hydrating, taking breaks, getting a footrest – and make a few small changes to your work routine. For starters, inform everyone around you that your due date is close. If your place of work has a strict dress code, speak to someone about making an allowance. You may need those comfy flats and breathable clothes. You may need more breaks to visit the toilet and stretch your legs and sit more often if your work requires long hours on your feet. You may need relaxation aids (like warm packs or a back pillow). See if you can take a day off once in a while. Perhaps you could figure out an arrangement to work shorter hours a day or fewer days a week.

Can I drive my car?

Women all over the world drive their own cars throughout their pregnancy. There is no more danger in driving a car when you're pregnant than at any other given time! A lot of pregnant mums find a few tips helpful (and comfortable) when they're driving: (1) Wear your seatbelt properly – the lap belt goes under your abdomen (as low as possible) and the shoulder belt goes between the breasts. Keep it snug. (2) Don't sit terribly close to the steering wheel. Check if your feet reach the pedals comfortably and if your knees can bend a little bit. (3) When you're very big, if you have the option of getting driven by someone else, take it! (4) And, needless to say, drive slow and steady so you don't experience any sudden jerks when braking.

Will I hurt my baby if I push on my stomach?

Your baby is really well cushioned in there! You can massage your belly gently. You can allow someone else to touch it, though only if you don't mind. What is scary is if you fall flat right on your belly, or if your belly gets pushed very hard. You should definitely speak to your doctor and opt for a Nonstress Test (NST) in this case. If your older kid gives you a squishy belly hug or throws a ball against your belly, you needn't panic (it happens to everyone!).

Can I still get a massage?

Yes, a massage can work wonders with relieving tension, aches, stress and swelling. But it would be best to follow the same cautions as we outlined earlier in trimester two. As a rule of thumb, stay safe by avoiding all the pressure points (i.e., reflexology areas) associated with your wrist, foot, hands, ankles and pelvis. You can always opt for a relaxing casual massage by your partner or a friend or a certified prenatal massage therapist. A relaxing and soothing back massage can be given to you till the very end of term – even while you're in labour.

What can't I do?

Let's address the common questions.

Can I carry my kid while I'm pregnant?

You shouldn't be carrying anything heavy especially in trimester three but you may not often have a choice with a toddler in tow! Avoid it as much as possible and really try and be strict by the end. If you have to, hold your kid on your hip (sideways), and under your bump. When you pick him up, it is best not to bend down from your waist. Bend your knees a little and lift with your legs. If you are breathless, spotting, feeling pain, have a backache, at risk of preterm labour or have conditions like placenta previa (PP) or short cervix, your doctor will advise you against carrying your older kid at any point in your pregnancy.

The pregnancy posture FAQs

With your bump at max, it's worthwhile to pay a bit of attention to your posture during this trimester. The golden rule when you're pregnant is to place minimal strain on your back when you walk, exercise, sleep, sit or stand. So, it helps to change positions every 30 minutes. Be mindful to stand with equal pressure on both your feet, keeping them hip-distance apart and with your back neutral rather than arched in.

1. **What position can I sleep in?**
    The stomach is out. And while there is no definitive research on sleeping on your back, it is generally not recommended and is eventually avoidable because the entire weight of your growing belly rests on your back, vena cava and intestines. That leaves you with but one choice: sleeping on your side. On an average, pregnant women are encouraged to sleep on their left side although both sides are okay. Why the left? Lying on your left is also recommended in yoga! It is meant to improve circulation to the heart, keep the pressure off your liver and allow proper blood flow. Refer back to the sleeping pillows we discussed in trimester two, in case you're feeling nervous about hurting your baby while you sleep.

2. **Will I squish my baby by bending over?**
    Your baby is really safe in there – well cushioned in amniotic fluid and your uterus. Bending down to pick something up off the floor is not going to harm your baby but it may make you uncomfortable. Your back is sensitive enough without you adding pressure to it. Pregnant or not, fitness pros will always advice us to pick something from the floor by

centring our core, bending our hips and knees and lowering our body straight. When pregnant, grip something close to you to help you stand back up, if you need it. When rising up from a chair, it's better to slide forward and stand (rather than bend from the waist).

3. **Can I cross my legs when I sit? Can I sit cross-legged on the floor?**

    Experts say you must sit with your back well supported, and try and place equal pressure on both your hips. This is why it is better to sit on a chair with both feet planted on the ground in front of you, rather than to cross your legs. In many cases, pregnant women find it hard to cross their legs. For women who are dealing with pelvic girdle issues of any form, varicose veins, leg swelling or weight issues, sitting cross-legged on the floor is definitely avoidable. But for most women it is absolutely okay to sit cross-legged on the floor, as long as you're comfortable.

What happens at the doctor's?

From 29 weeks up until you reach 36 weeks, your doctor will see you every two weeks. Post this time, you will be seeing your doctor every week. As mentioned earlier, this schedule will vary by a few extra appointments for concerns, queries, scares, follow-ups or as required if you are carrying multiple babies.

Your vaccine schedule has most likely been wrapped up in trimester two. Do check with your doctor if he/she prefers to administer the tetanus shot in the last trimester, at 30–32 weeks, instead of in the second trimester. You will be doing routine ultrasounds, blood tests and urine tests through trimester three.

What will your doctor be looking for? There will of course be your weight and blood pressure. Some doctors check and measure your bump. Later, your cervix may be examined for signs of dilation. Your urine tests are important to gauge the presence of infections as well as proteins and sugars that are indicative of pre-eclampsia and gestational diabetes. In case you have a history of anaemia, you will be asked for a blood test.

This is the time to speak to your doctor about the pain relief options available to you during childbirth. Think about whether you prefer an episiotomy or natural tearing during a vaginal birth (see Chapter 4: Labour and Childbirth to understand more on your pain relief options during a vaginal birth and also about episiotomy versus natural tearing). There is no decisive answer to the episiotomy question; it depends on your preference or on what your ob-gyn recommends. Clear your doubts on forceps or vacuum assistance during a normal delivery. Discuss the odds of a Caesarean birth. Talk to your doctor about any changes or symptoms you may be experiencing that concern you.

Note: If you are keen on 3D/4D scans, the further you go past 34 weeks, the tougher the chances of achieving proper images, owing to the slowly decreasing fluid levels around the baby and the baby's own rapidly growing body. If you are lucky and the sonologist finds your baby in a favourable position with fluid around the face, you will be able to get an amazing picture of your baby, complete with features and expressions.

What tests will I need to take?

Between 35 and 38 weeks: GBS screen or Group B Streptococcus Screening is done for the group B strep bacteria that exist in our bowels, rectum, bladder, vagina and throat. It is a significant but preventable cause of poor maternal and infant health worldwide. A 2017 study by the London School of Hygiene & Tropical Medicine, UK, revealed that one in five pregnant women globally carried the GBS bacteria, with India ranking the highest. Rather than screening based on risk, doctors in India follow a policy of universal GBS screening. This bacteria can cause potentially dangerous infections in newborn babies. An immediate course of antibiotics is recommended for moms who test positive for this bacteria. The test entails two cotton swab samples taken from the lower vagina and rectum.

Blood tests (once, to be repeated if needed)
- CBC – for infections
- HIV, HCV – for HIV and Hepatitis C virus
- HbsAg – Hepatitis B surface antigen, to check for the Hepatitis B virus
- Random blood sugar – to check your blood glucose level
- Creatinine – measures your creatinine, which reflects how your kidneys are working. While this test is optional, it is always safer to do it once before delivery

Urine test (once, to be repeated if needed)
- Urine routine test and urine protein test

NST (only if required)
The nonstress test is performed towards the end of term to check on the baby as needed. In high-risk pregnancies or multiple babies, this test can start weekly from 28 weeks or is usually done twice a week towards the end of term or as often as needed (even daily) before birth. Most Indian doctors will recommend

an NST for you if you are overdue, or if your baby isn't moving normally or for any other concerns. An NST can have a reactive or non-reactive result. In case of the latter, there are further tests your doctor may suggest, like an NST combined with an ultrasonography and Doppler.

Doppler study (once, if required; to be repeated if required)
This is to keep track of the circulation of blood in the baby, the uterus, placenta and umbilical artery for your doctor to be able to assess any adverse outcomes related to your delivery and to the baby's health. This test can be conducted by your sonologist, your doctor or a technician who is trained in ultrasound imaging. The process is the same as an ultrasound: a gel will be applied on your bare abdomen and a transducer will be moved across the area to get images. You are asked to get a Doppler study after 28 weeks to assess foetal circulation and utero-placental circulation.

A breakdown of your third trimester ultrasounds

During my second pregnancy, I did involve Taimur and always showed him my ultrasound scans, especially the lovely 3D pictures given to us by Dr Mitossh. Taimur may not have understood exactly what was being shown to him. But it was a great way to prepare him for the arrival of his sibling.

It is important to check foetal growth and health, the baby's position, cervix and amniotic fluid. There are moms who voluntarily choose to get an ultrasound every week from around 37 weeks till they deliver.

At 30 weeks: A routine ultrasound to monitor foetal growth and all the other parameters. For multiple babies, your doctor may recommend an NST along with the ultrasound at this stage.

Around 36 weeks: A routine foetal well-being scan and most likely a colour Doppler foetal examination.

At 38 weeks: A colour Doppler foetal examination and a foetal biophysical profile.

(With inputs from Dr Mitossh Ruparel)

What medicines do I need?

Here's a little caveat. No drug can be considered 100 per cent safe to use during pregnancy. Beyond a basic paracetamol, most moms do not consume any medicines without consulting with their doctor. The same rules apply as discussed in trimesters one and two. Your regular prenatal vitamins and supplements are safe, effective and critical till the very last day. Your doctor may choose to put you on medication for BP or sugar, if you need it. Just in case you have a known history of preterm labour or are at a high risk for premature delivery, your doctor may give you hydroxyprogesterone injections any time post the 16–20-week mark until the time you deliver. This will help lower the risk of giving birth too early.

Complications of trimester three

Can we skip the scary stuff, you might be thinking as we come to this section. It's true, complications can be scary, but staying in the know will help equip you and alert you to the potential red flags. So take a deep breath and read on!

As was the case in trimesters one and two, heavy bleeding at any time in your pregnancy is a big red flag. Most of the list of pregnancy complications remains the same as before: **pre-**

eclampsia, placenta previa, gestational diabetes, pregnancy-induced hypertension, cervical incompetence, preterm labour and **PPROM**.

However, there are certain other complications that can arise during this time. If the baby does not settle into a head down (i.e., vertex) position towards the end of trimester three, it is known as **malpresentation** and it is when the baby is either sideways (transverse) or head up (breech). A severe body itch called **obstetric cholestasis** – without the appearance of any rash – is another issue that may crop up in trimester three.

A very rare and grave complication is **placental abruption**, where the placenta separates from the uterus before labour. Foetal distress, back pain, cramps, hardening of the uterus and serious vaginal bleeding can occur in these cases. Medical intervention needs to be very swift. Another uncommon and serious risk is **placental insufficiency**, when the placenta fails to deliver adequate nutrients to the foetus. It can be identified only by a drop in the baby's movements or through an NST or ultrasound. **Intrauterine growth restriction (IUGR)** is another situation that can come about when the baby doesn't grow as much as expected. IUGR babies need to be monitored very closely and are delivered by 37 weeks. IUGR babies mostly will not be able to withstand normal labour, hence the chances of a Caesarean delivery are high.

If pregnancy stretches beyond 40 weeks or more, it is called **post-term** and is risky. Why? Beyond about 41 weeks, the placenta's function is compromised, the umbilical cord can compress and the amniotic fluid also may decrease significantly. Post-term pregnancies have to be monitored closely as the risk of meconium aspiration and intrauterine death is high. As mentioned earlier, amniotic fluid peaks at around 35 weeks and then gradually decreases. But if it gets too low it is called **oligohydramnios** and if it gets too high it is called **polyhydramnios** – both are considered complications. Both these phenomena are diagnosed by ultrasonography measurements of amniotic fluid volume.

While we have gone over many serious pregnancy issues over trimesters one and two, there are some terms which still need to be explored in detail.

What does a 'low-lying placenta' even mean?

This is a term you have heard earlier through trimester one and trimester two and is something that you will encounter frequently. Basically, a low-lying placenta or **placenta previa** (PP) is when the placenta is in the lower part of your uterus, thereby obstructing your cervix – which is the 'outlet' for the uterus (i.e., the place for the baby to exit your uterus into the birth canal). In the normal course of things, a complication-free placenta is located at the top of the uterus or, at most, at the side of the uterus.

Now, PP can occur in three ways: (1) **complete or total PP**: when the placenta is fully obstructing/covering the cervix – which means there is no option but a Caesarean birth; (2) **partial PP**: when the edge of the placenta is partly covering the cervix – so a normal vaginal delivery may not work out; (3) **marginal PP**: when the placenta is adjacent to the cervix – in this case, a normal vaginal delivery is possible.

While PP will be identifiable during trimesters one and two, the reason it is mentioned in detail at trimester three is that both partial PP and marginal PP may move away from the cervix as your pregnancy advances. But if you have a form of PP till late in your pregnancy, it may have implications like preterm delivery or a Caesarean birth.

Apart from PP, there are two other rarer forms of placental placements that are considered just a little out of the ordinary: (1) **anterior placenta**: when it attaches to the front, i.e., near your stomach; (2) **posterior placenta**: when it attaches to the back, i.e., near your spine. Bear in mind that an anterior placenta means you are a little cushioned from feeling your baby's kicks very strongly.

How does PP impact your pregnancy? Well, if you have had a form of PP from trimester one, you're likely to have been bleeding a little bit throughout your pregnancy. Your doctor will monitor your placenta placement from your first trimester. While PP does not have an impact on the health of the baby during the nine months, it can cause excess bleeding during labour and birth. Why? It is because your cervix begins to thin out anyway for the process of labour. The blood vessels between the placenta and uterus may begin to tear too. PP can lead to torrential bleeding in many cases, causing BP to drop and necessitating hospital/ICU care. An emergency C-section or a blood transfusion are possible outcomes.

Uncontrollable itching? It could be obstetric cholestasis

There are times when this itch can manifest earlier in a pregnancy, but most women who have dealt with it report it most commonly during trimester three. It is not a very commonly occurring problem and is a form of intense itching that comes out of nowhere (your body doesn't have a rash), is more pronounced on the palms and soles and is often worse at night. It could also be everywhere. With this, your urine may appear dark and your stool lighter in colour and smelly. Most often, this itchiness fixes itself post delivery. Why does it happen? There is no certain answer. It could be genetic/hereditary or because as your pregnancy hormones slow down, the flow of bile from your liver that is meant to exit your system instead builds up in it, thereby causing the bile salts to enter your bloodstream and make you itchy. You will have to speak to your doctor about this. What your doctor is likely to do is: (a) run some blood tests for bile acid and enzymes, (b) check you for signs of jaundice, (c) ask for an ultrasound, (d) give you medication and recommend a few lifestyle changes and (e) in an extreme case, a liver biopsy is recommended, and you may be sent to a hepatologist for a consultation.

What is a stillbirth?

As per the WHO, the loss of a baby before 28 weeks of pregnancy is termed a miscarriage. But beyond this period, it is called a stillbirth. A stillborn baby is one that displays no sign of life and has died in vitro during pregnancy, labour or birth. There may be multiple causes for stillbirth, like placental problems, pre-eclampsia, infection, lifestyle choices, trauma, clotting disorders, birth defects and more. Despite the progress in prenatal care, stillbirths still occur and many stillbirths cannot even be explained. At 20 to 27 weeks, it is an 'early' stillbirth and from 28 to 36 weeks, it is either a 'late' or 'term' stillbirth.

The symptoms of a possible stillbirth are complete lack of foetal movement; cramping and vaginal spotting/bleeding may also occur. Sadly, some stillbirths can go unnoticed for weeks as there are no tangible manifestations. The only sure way to confirm a stillbirth is through an ultrasound and/or Doppler scan. In case of most stillbirths, the ob-gyn induces labour and recommends a vaginal delivery of the baby.

It takes four to six weeks for the body to heal post a stillbirth and return to normal. But emotionally, coming to terms with a stillborn baby at any point of time in your pregnancy will be heartbreaking. Most parents of stillborn babies choose to commemorate their baby with a funeral and a prayer. Take your time with processing this loss. You may not feel normal for a while. Rely on the support of your friends, family and even a counsellor to work through your grief.

Preparations for trimester three

I admit I am one of those highly prepared people—I am very organized. My family has always been superstitious, so I didn't buy a thing until my seventh month. But during my seventh and eighth months, I got ready for my babies. This happened both times. I shopped for the babies myself and got their nurseries ready. And I kept my hospital bag packed and ready before I reached 38 weeks.

Shall I go shopping now?

This is the time to go shopping for your post-delivery needs and your baby and nursery supplies (see Part III: Getting Ready for the Baby: Your Definitive Guide to Shopping and Planning for the Nursery).

Should I pack my hospital bag?

Yes! Unless you're expecting twins, who are likelier to birth early, you should keep your hospital bag ready by the 37-week mark.

You'll be surprised by how calming this process can be for you (see section 'What do I pack in my hospital bag?').

Update your medical file with absolutely all your ultrasound and blood reports, hospital receipts/registration, birthing notes and other research. Also keep the numbers of your emergency contacts, ob-gyn and paediatrician handy. Make sure your partner and/or family members also have the numbers of your ob-gyn and paediatrician handy.

Who will my baby's paediatrician be?

A paediatrician will always be present during the birth of your baby; i.e., it will be a doctor who is affiliated with the hospital you are giving birth at. If there are multiple doctors available, you can request a specific one for your delivery – of course, during the time of birth, if your pre-selected paediatrician cannot make it, another doctor will be present. You may decide to stick with the hospital's empanelled paediatrician long term. If the doctor meets your criteria of requirements of a paediatrician, you can continue by all means to remain in his/her care. However, you can also move to another paediatrician after you've been discharged from the hospital, for all subsequent baby care. If you are going with a pre-selected paediatrician, make sure you also call him/her when you're headed to the hospital, or have your hospital call the doctor for you. The paediatrician will be in the operation theatre with your ob-gyn when you give birth.

Use your time in trimester three to zero in on a paediatrician for your baby and get an appointment to go meet him/her in advance. Your paediatrician and you will be raising this baby after all, and it is important you find a doctor who is on the same page as you, with whom you can share an equation of trust and understanding. This is the doctor in whom you will be putting all your faith. Pick a doctor who is affiliated to a proper hospital if possible, so things are easier in case of any emergencies. Try and look for someone in your vicinity. As a matter of fact, the American Academy of Pediatrics (AAP) recommends scheduling a prenatal visit to the paediatrician – just so you can discuss your pregnancy and health, medical complications, baby immunizations and so on. You'll be surprised at how many years your kid may choose to visit his/her paediatrician (yes, even at 21!).

If your ob-gyn is very particular, he/she may consult your paediatrician from early in your pregnancy (even from 26–32 weeks) if you have complications. This could be for reasons like preterm labour preparation, administering any steroids and so on. More and more urban Indian paediatricians recommend that you have this meeting before you give birth. If you have a normal, complication-free pregnancy, see if you can have this meeting before 37 weeks.

Preparing your kid for the arrival of a sibling

Timing is very important. The start of your third trimester may be the best time to introduce your pregnancy to your older kid or kids. The 28-week mark is especially important for kids who are younger than four or five because it is otherwise extraordinarily difficult for them to process that the baby is 'not coming' – in case of any mishap. As we've discussed earlier in this book, a baby born post the 28-week mark, even premature, has an excellent chance of survival.

Start by laying out the bare facts – that there is a baby in your tummy and he is going to be a new addition to the family. If your first child is still young, books are a wonderful way to introduce the concept of a new baby and a sibling. There are lovely books available – for older and younger kids. Get online or speak to friends and find interesting book titles that work for you. Talk about babies and what babies are like, what they need, what they do. Get some baby name suggestions from them. Take him/her shopping for the baby. Should you take your older kid for an ultrasound appointment? Speak to your sonologist about it. It is ideal to wait till your eighth month for this. It is great to keep up an honest, chatty conversation about the new baby.

Before the birth of your baby, put up photographs of your older child at birth, getting a massage, being cuddled, being bathed, at his/her naming ceremony and so on. It is important for them to see that they were just as loved and cared for as the coming baby is going to be.

Let your older child feel a sense of ownership: like this is his/her baby! Before birth and for at least 15 to 20 days post delivery, address this baby as 'your baby' when you speak to your older kid (or 'X's baby brother' or 'X's baby sister' when you speak to other people). Let X be of primary importance! Tell your family and your friends to do the same. Any gifts that come for your baby should be handed over to your older kid – 'this is for you for having a baby' is a lovely thing for them to hear. It is important for your child to feel secure about this new arrival. Remember, your newborn has no concept of gifts or attention, but your older kid understands all of it.

A tip to keep in mind for when you deliver the baby: keep a little gift ready for your older child, and this is especially relevant if your kid is still young. When they first see the baby (either at the hospital or when you come back home), give it to them and tell them it is a gift from the baby.

Now, about the time you will spend nursing your new baby! Towards the end of your third trimester, start speaking about animal babies with your older kid. Especially talk about how all babies feed from their mothers. Feel free to share photos of a breastfeeding mom too. And when your new baby is home, address all of your older kid's curiosity surrounding breastfeeding. Rather than sending them out of your room and locking yourself in and telling them 'it's private', let them sit with you and read a book or chat or just watch. Express a couple of drops of breast milk and show it to them. Let it be as natural as having a cup of tea. Tell them the baby is drinking milk because he doesn't have teeth. Tell them that they did the same when they were born. Almost every kid under about three and a half years will ask their moms for a taste. Say yes. Every mom who has been through this has said that their kid will take one sniff or make one attempt and then promptly lose interest and run off. Hopefully, all those desperate and heartbreaking knocks at your door will stop!

(With inputs from Dr Neeru Vithalani)

How I prepared my son for the arrival of his sibling

Taimur is a very social, warm, confident and friendly kid. He loves other children. Saif's sister Soha's daughter Inaaya is pretty much his sibling! She is with him all the time. He loves people around the house. Whether it was our family or friends, we have always had people over. We are a busy home, bustling with eaters and drinkers. And Taimur was always a part of it. He would be playing Lego on the floor as we caught up with our friends. It was never about 'not involving kids' or sending him away. But yes, he kept to his bedtime routine strictly! I truly believe that parents who are inclusive raise confident kids. I introduced the subject to Taimur by explaining to him that he came from my tummy. That there was now another life there and that he would soon have a baby brother or sister. I asked him how he felt about it. He was very excited. He was never upset about it. He wasn't insecure. And I credit a large part of that to Saif. He is an incredibly hands-on dad. That's what keeps Taimur so secure. What he missed was me carrying him. He loves being carried and cuddled – though now he towers over me when I carry him. Throughout my pregnancy, he would ask me a single question: 'When the baby comes out, will you carry me?' I couldn't carry him for a long time. But when I felt my Caesarean stitches had healed enough after Jeh, I picked him up. And he ran to tell his father excitedly. He sees me carrying Jeh around now. So I have to carry him too. He is thrilled and excited about having a little brother. In two months, he read him three stories. He lies in bed with him and asks me why Jeh won't play with him. He is already talking about all the bank robber games he will play with him. He knows what stories he is going to tell him. He is all heart. He does not have any sibling rivalry because we have never allowed him to feel less important, even for a minute.

What is cord blood banking?

Cord blood banking is a process in which you can register and pay a stem cell bank to preserve your baby's cord blood on a private basis for a duration of 21 years. What's cord blood? Once the baby is born, the umbilical cord is cut and clamped. The 75–150 ml of cord blood collected from it contains stem cells which can be used in the future for stem cell therapy and its related diseases. It's painless for the mother and baby. It is transported to the cord banking facility and stored in a frozen state. The mother's blood is screened for a variety of diseases too. This process starts in trimester three when you zero in on a stem cell bank that services your city. You pay for yearly or lifetime storage in advance. Representatives may visit you at home for a demonstration, to explain the process. Your doctor and hospital should be informed of your arrangement too.

The statistics of cord blood storage in India are still very low. Worldwide, there is not enough scientific data yet that indicates any major advantages to private cord blood banking. Again, this is a personal decision and is not mandatory. Nor does it have any sweeping implications on the future health of your baby. Understand the cost versus the viability and talk to your doctor and paediatrician before you make a decision about storing cord blood for your baby. Many doctors may tell you to instead donate the stem cells to a publicly accessible cord blood bank.

It is best to discuss cord blood banking with your paediatrician in advance as he/she will be present at the birth of your baby. This is because delayed cord clamping is now standard protocol at childbirth (see box 'What is DCC?'), so the cord blood continues to flow to your baby. It is ideally done for about five minutes post birth, till the cord pulsation stops. A little cord blood may be left over thereafter for cord blood banking.

Some moms start massaging their breasts in trimester three: What is that about?

This is a little pre-lactation trick that prenatal experts recommend, post the 37–38-week mark: do a short daily breast massage for yourself using any oil or moisturizer. Simply place four fingers of each hand on the same breast (top and bottom) and follow a circular kneading pattern – about three to five circles. Doing so is said to prevent stretch marks on the breast, and dry and cracked nipples during breastfeeding, and to encourage the process of lactation.

Perineum massage – it sounds crazy!

Many women globally choose to do this post their 36-week mark, in preparation for a vaginal birth. Your perineum is the little area between your vagina and anus. Prenatal and birthing experts and pregnant women say a perineum massage reduces your chances of having an episiotomy. It is likely your ob-gyn will recommend you commence this massage on yourself. How do you do this massage? Sit well supported (preferably in front of a mirror in the beginning) with your legs apart. Use two fingers, dipped in extra virgin olive oil, and rub along the area. Move outwards (centre to sides) and downwards (in to out). Do this every day, for 15–20 seconds initially and go up to four to five minutes.

Looking up Lamaze

This is a controlled breathing practice based on the idea of helping women in labour relax to ease their pain. It comprises slow deep breaths in different rhythms – mainly a combination of 'hee' inhalations and 'hoo' exhalations from the mouth. A lot of women practise Lamaze breathing and many manage to successfully exercise their Lamaze breathing during childbirth too. While there are no statistics on Lamaze practice in India, Lamaze lessons are available in many pockets of urban India, through prenatal consultants, hospitals/birthing centres or private clinics. Most moms take Lamaze classes or begin their Lamaze practice sometime during the third trimester – the seventh month would work.

(With inputs from Dr Neeru Vithalani and Dr Rita Shah)

Packing your hospital bag

During both my pregnancies, I was prepared with my hospital bag by the time I completed 37 weeks. I would recommend you do so too. Just like any other first-time mom, I too looked up all the must-have lists of essentials and tried to use them as a guide for my hospital bag. I read about how many women pack their music and scented candles. But in my head I thought: how will I have time for any of it?! I had no music, massage ball or room scents! Instead, I packed a bunch of sanitary napkins, big-sized cotton underwear, napkins, clothes for the hospital and a set of clothes to come home in. You know what was the most important thing I packed? Five cotton nursing bras from Marks & Spencer. And, oh, towels! I am very particular about my own hand, face and body towels. I packed a simple baby set with a single onesie, diaper and swaddle to bring Taimur home in. It was a hand-me-down. For Jeh, I carried one set of Taimur's old baby clothes to come home in. Don't they say babies should come home in old clothes?

While there is no fixed time to keep your hospital bag packed and ready, most moms (who have had a healthy pregnancy, are having singleton babies and expecting to go full term) will keep their bag ready by week 36–37. If you're expecting to give birth sooner, then be prepared in advance. You'll be surprised at how calm it will make you feel. Bear in mind, it is best to leave all your valuables at home. You have enough to worry about as it is. Keep this list as a broad-spectrum checklist of everything you may possibly need. Except for a few snacks, your cell phone, chargers and some last-minute comfortable pants, there is no reason for 95 per cent of this bag not to be packed in advance.

1. One cute baby outfit to bring the baby home in from the hospital – for all those photo-ops! This set should include a ganji, swaddle cloth, cap and a 'receiving blanket' (optional). Your baby will be in hospital-issued garments and diapers till he is ready to go. You could carry two diapers for your baby. You can borrow baby clothes from friends or family too

2. One outfit for you to go home in

3. Your hospital file – with all pregnancy reports, blood work, ultrasounds. Your notes on Lamaze, labour and other tips you've been gathering

4. A sweater, shawl, or jacket – in case you get cold

5. If you're fussy about your own linen – carry your own towel. There is a chance you may be sponged until your doctor switches your Caesarean incision to a waterproof dressing and clears you to shower. In case of a vaginal birth, you can shower normally

6. Carry your own bath products if you prefer. Remember the little things that bring you comfort, like your lip balm, moisturizer, deodorant, toothbrush, toothpaste, hairbrush, hair-ties/headbands. In case you're nuts about washing your hair, carry a shampoo and a small hair dryer

7. Music and/or reading material. And, to make things super easy, download a few movies or shows on your gadget in advance – in case the labour goes on for a while

8. Your gadgets/cell phone and chargers with appropriate adapters. Take a camera, if you want to take more than cell phone pictures!

9. A pair of slippers for the hospital

10. After you slip out of your hospital gown post day one, you can wear your own clothes – so pack the button-down shirts and comfortable pants for day wear and nightclothes too. Always pack for about four days, just in case. Why? A C-section is usually followed by a four-day stay at the hospital

11. One packet of sanitary napkins (non-synthetic surfaces may really help in the beginning when you may be dealing with stitches). The hospital will provide surgical sanitary napkins for you

12. Three nursing bras and six large-sized cotton underwear minimum, as you may stain your underwear. Some moms pick up disposable maternity underwear for the hospital stay

13. A small make-up kit – optional; if you feel like

14. Some small dry snacks, candy, your favourite chocolate

15. A cheap clock with a seconds hand might be handy to time your contractions or use your cell phone timer

16. A pen and a notepad – for anything!

17. Your own breast pump, if you like

Your birthing partner should be prepared for a prolonged stay at the hospital for you, just in case. Here is what your partner should prep with:

- Chargers with appropriate adapters
- A file with the hospital registration receipt, health insurance card and paperwork, cash and credit cards
- Change of clothes
- A sweater, shawl, jumper or jacket – in case it gets cold
- A small dry snack, candy, chocolate
- A set of personal toiletries
- Music and/or reading

End of trimester three: Quick look

Baby: While every baby is different, most average full-term healthy babies weigh in at 2.5 kg to 3.5 kg – some going up to 4.5 kg. Most average full-term healthy babies measure about 18 to 22 inches. This little human is in your hands by the end of trimester three.

Mom: Your belly will be huge, and you will be about 11 to 15 kg up (on an average) or more. Apart from the weight of your baby, your uterus will be weighing in at 1 kg at the time of birth, your placenta at 0.7 kg and the amniotic fluid at 0.8 kg.

PART II

LABOUR AND CHILDBIRTH, AND WHAT COMES IMMEDIATELY AFTER

My countdown to the end

T hose final weeks till the big day are really something else! I was a bundle of nerves and found it hard to relax. And let me tell you, baby two doesn't make it easier. You would have thought that I was a seasoned hand by the time I was inching closer to Jeh's due date. But, no! There were so many nights I couldn't sleep, from my eighth month onwards. It happens to all of us, I guess. It is the anxiety, the excitement and who knows what else.

I didn't have too much mindspace to overthink things during Jeh's time. I had just about wrapped up my work commitments by my eighth month and – of course – I had Taimur to keep me busy. I was so active and so overworked with shoots and the house move that I would crash into deep dreamless sleep the minute my head hit the pillow. Of course, this only lasted a few hours. I would wake up suddenly in the middle of the night and spend the rest of the time tossing and turning. I am a back sleeper, so trying to stay on my side was torture.

But I tried to stay focused and calm by doing a little meditation for about fifteen minutes every day. It was nothing heavy duty.

I just made a little bit of time to be alone and tried to think positive thoughts. This was especially useful on the days when I felt anxious. I also rely heavily on yoga during my non-pregnant days. I find it really centres me.

My nesting instinct kicked in big time towards the end of my third trimester. I moved homes in a complete frenzy, and it helped that the new house was across the road. I'll admit it was rough and I probably pushed myself a little too hard. I felt heavy. My back gave way a lot. I was on my feet for hours and oversaw every little detail, returning home with aching legs and back. But I just had to get it done! Saif and I were really keen to settle into our new family home before the little one arrived.

I managed to fully move my home in just about 15 days – clothes, furniture, kitchen and all. In fact, my new house was spotlessly clean and completely unpacked and ready to use well before I delivered. I guess you have to do things yourself to really get them done well. By this time, I'll admit, I was raring for a massage! I have always been apprehensive about prenatal massages and never tried any. My doctor didn't allow them either. But I was already dreaming of the heavenly massages that I would soon have.

Every mother gets worried in the last few weeks – there are so many reasons. Tensions about the delivery, worries about what life is going to be like with the baby. If you are feeling stressed, I completely sympathize. I went through all those emotions. So many women do. In my second pregnancy, I had many bouts of crying and outbursts of emotions. Sometimes I felt aggressive. Sometimes I craved attention! I caught myself becoming ratty and impatient with Taimur and snappy with Saif or my mom. I felt terrible about it later but I also couldn't completely control these mood swings.

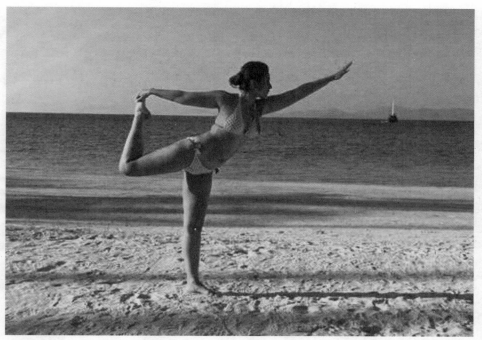

April 2016, Koh Samui. Yoga on the beach. I was pregnant with Taimur but didn't know it, and would only find out when I got back to Mumbai.

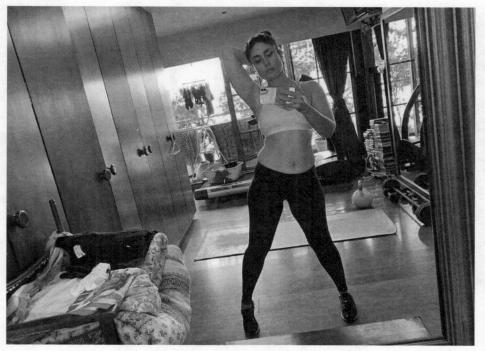

Here I am in June 2020. I didn't know I was pregnant with Jeh and would discover it only a few days later – though with him, I just knew another baby was on the way as soon as the symptoms hit.

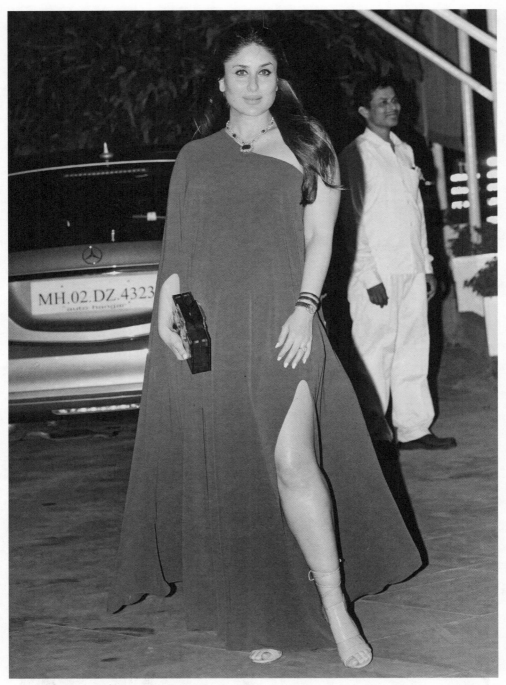

I had a wonderful pregnancy with Taimur – maybe it was my age.
I stayed up late, travelled, went to parties and felt great. This is one of
my all-time favourite pregnancy outfits.

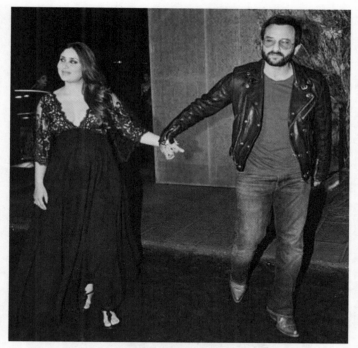

I was out and about all through my pregnancy. Two weeks after this evening out, I gave birth to Taimur!

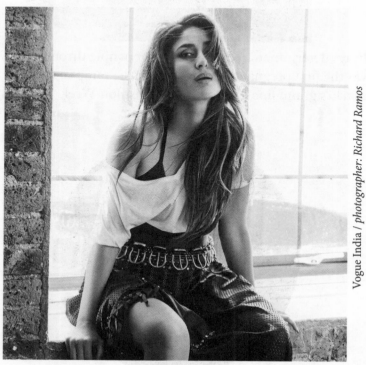

I did this shoot with *Vogue* in London, 4 months pregnant with Taimur. No one in the shoot knew I was expecting.

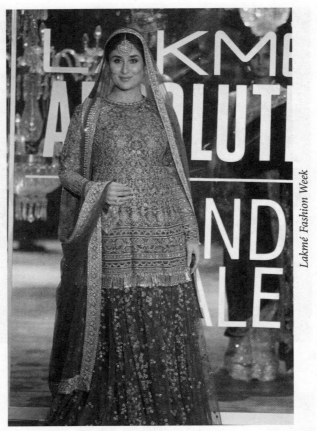

I was always determined to do as much as possible through the 9 months and was the first pregnant actress to walk the ramp in India. It was for Sabyasachi's grand finale at the Lakmé Fashion Week. I was 6 months gone with Taimur.

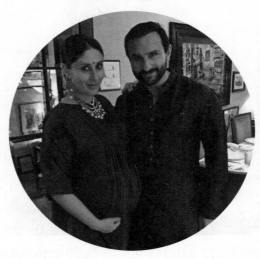

Diwali 2016 with Saif: I am 8 months pregnant with Taimur.

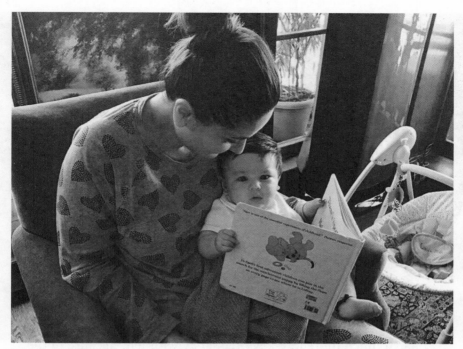

It took me a while to learn to handle Taimur when he was born. Like all new moms I was nervous and messed up all the time!

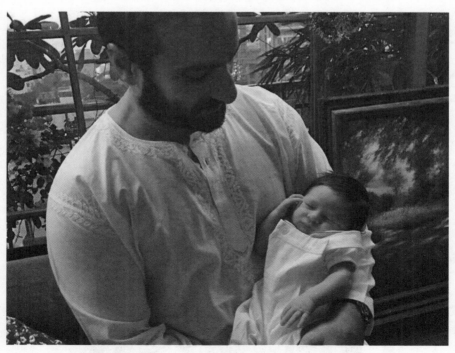

Saif, on the other hand, was much more confident in the early days! He tells me that I am very different with Jeh, much calmer!

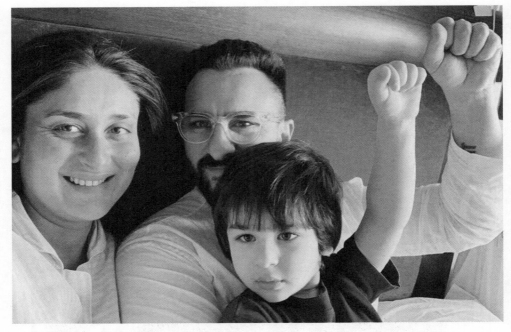

I had a much more low-key pregnancy with Jeh. Because of the
lockdown I was mostly at home with family or friends or at work.
Here we are on New Year's Day, bringing in 2021.

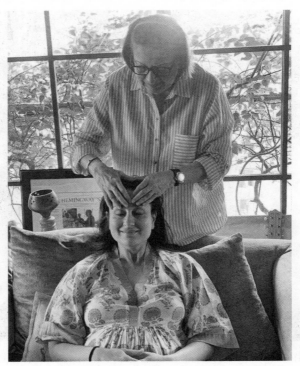

Mom giving me a relaxing head rub when I was pregnant with Jeh.
Just what every girl needs!

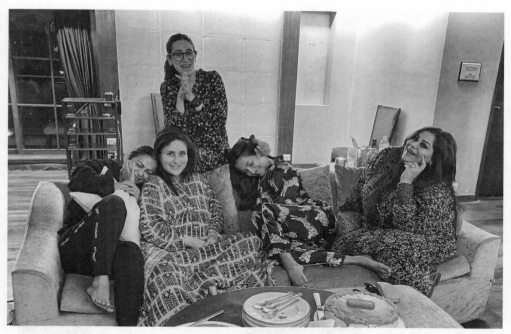

With my girl gang having a night-in at 8 months. This was the
last night we spent in our old flat.

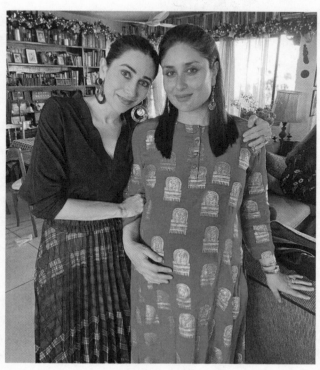

Christmas Day, 7.5 months pregnant with Jeh, with my beloved sister.

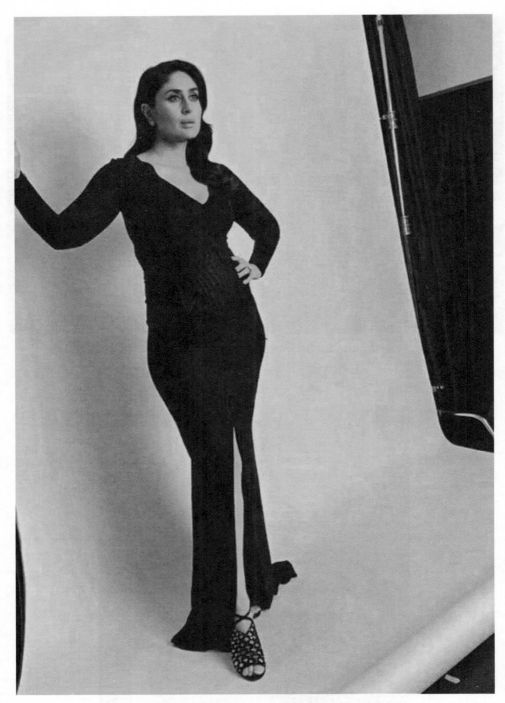

Unlike my first pregnancy, I was sick for the first trimester battling crazy nausea and had to manage exhaustion and low BP through a lot of the pregnancy. But unless it was an especially bad day, I continued working. Here I am doing a brand shoot, about 4 months with Jeh.

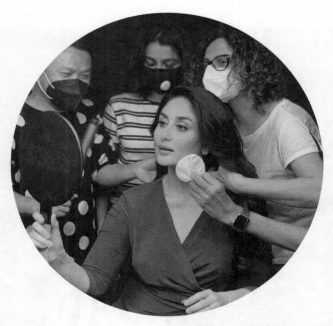

I did this shoot, pregnant, tired, bang in the middle of the lockdown!

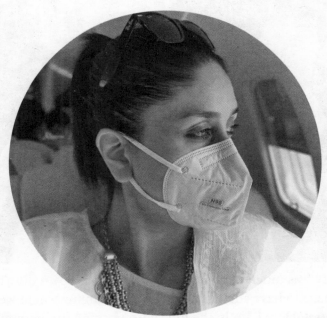

Flying to Delhi, during lockdown, for the *Laal Singh Chaddha* shoot. I was nervous flying in the middle of the pandemic, but was keen to finish my work before the baby came.

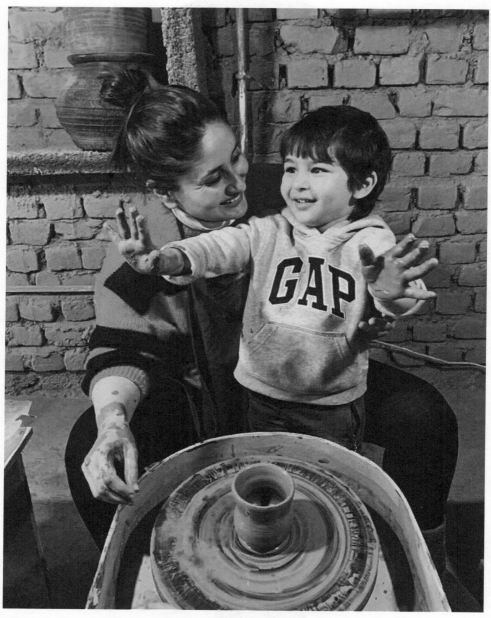

Jeh's pregnancy was much harder on me and the lockdown didn't help, but we did manage to have a few breaks like in Palampur where we joined Saif on a shoot. Here I am in the hill station having fun with my little guy.

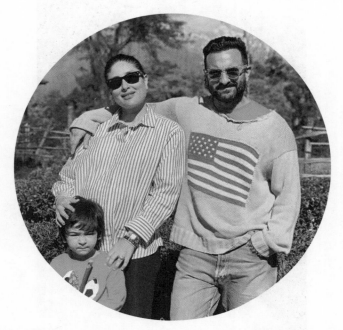

The getaway was exactly what I needed – I felt energized by the fresh mountain air. I was often tired and a bit anxious during this pregnancy and Saif and Taimur were really my biggest supports.

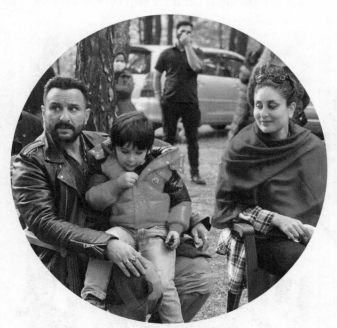

On the sets with Saif in Palampur.

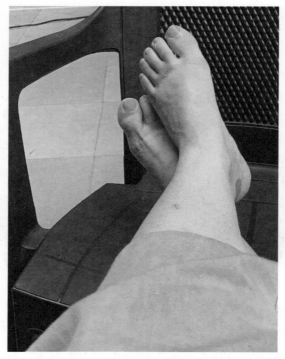

I found shooting for *Laal Singh Chaddha* really hard and would collapse in bed as soon as I finished my shoot. Here I am putting my swollen, tired feet up on the sets.

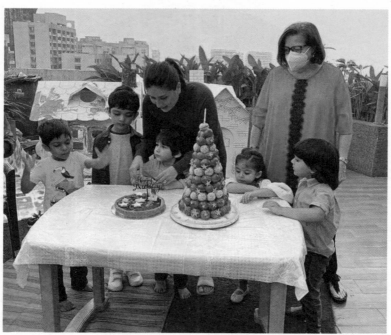

Taimur's birthday in 2020. I had just finished my radio show and came straight to the party.

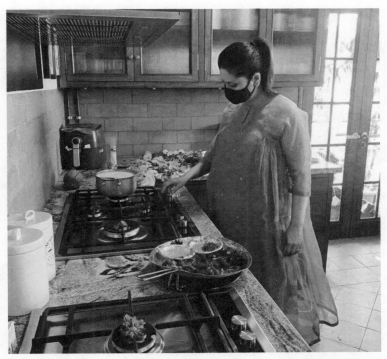

Doing a griha pravesh for our new flat. I was 8 months pregnant.

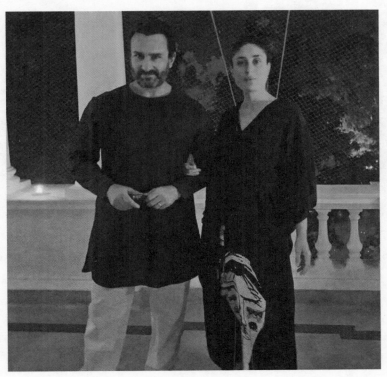

5 months pregnant with Jeh in Pataudi Palace. I lived in kaftans
through this pregnancy both day and night!

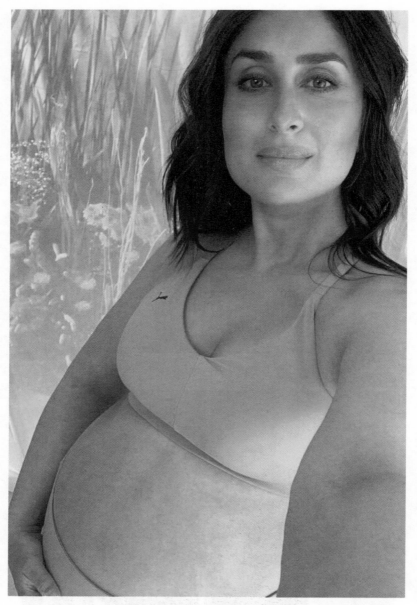

7 months pregnant with Jeh. I had gained a lot of weight but was comfortable with it and happy in my skin. When Puma asked me to do this shoot, I was game.

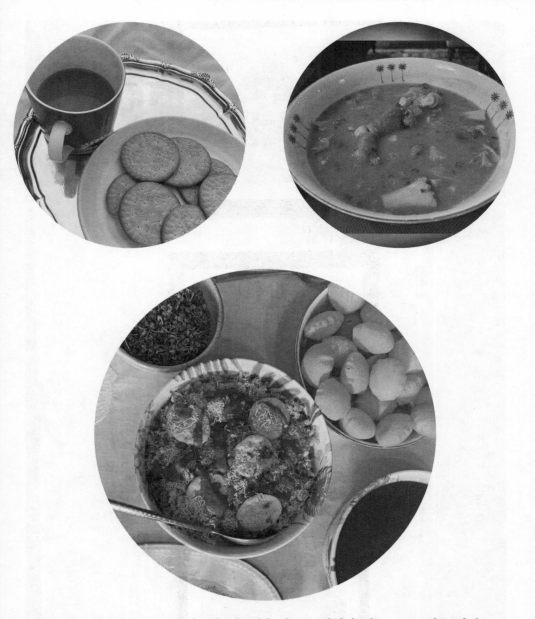

My pregnancy diet: I tried to be healthy but it didn't always work! I did try to keep my caffeine intake limited and would have only half a cup of tea (*top left*). Although not usually a chaat girl, I had massive chaat cravings (*bottom*) and, I have to admit, I frequently gave in! Through the 9 months, I swore by a home-made paya soup (*top right*) which is both delicious and nutritious.

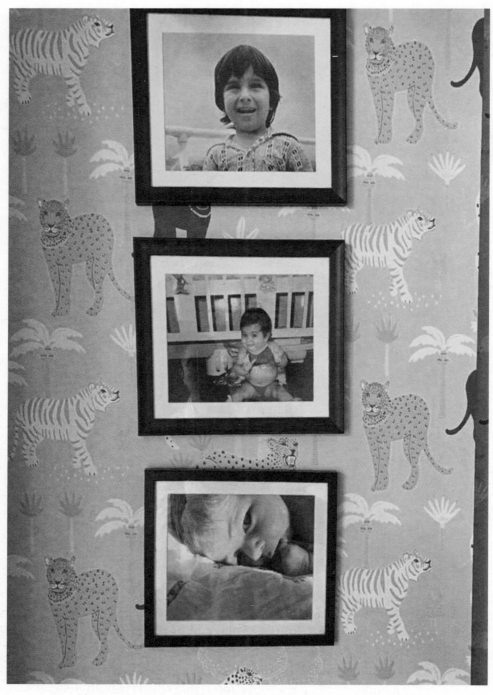

Jeh's nursery is one of my favourite rooms in our new flat.
We have pictures of Taimur, Saif and me as babies hung up on the wall.
Can you guess who is who?

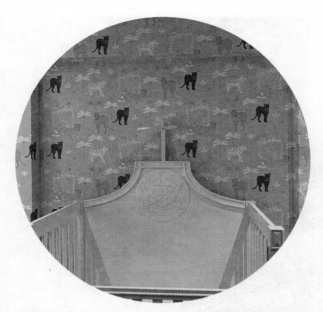

We built a special crib for Taimur with the Pataudi crest when he was born, which Jeh now uses.

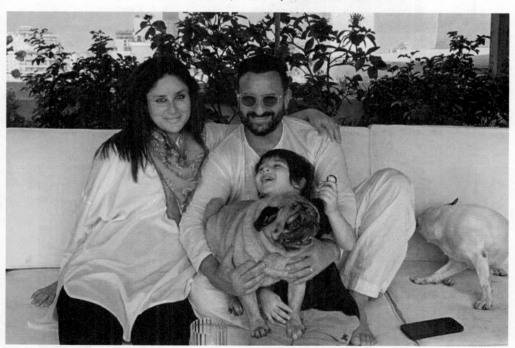

In the balcony in our new flat, two weeks before Jeh was born.

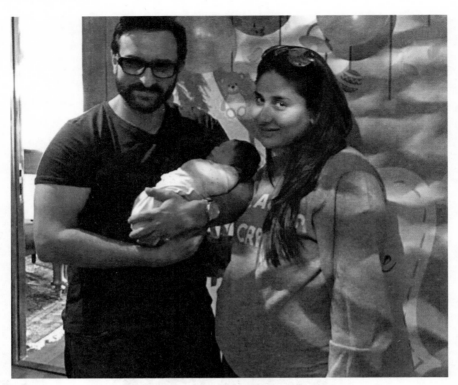

The day we brought Taimur home.

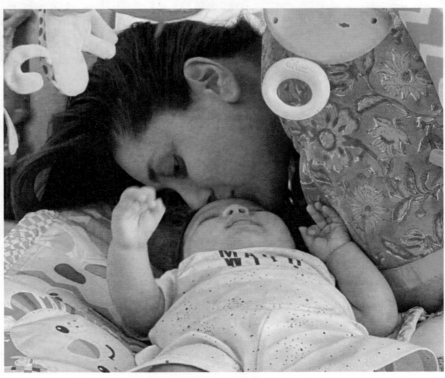

With my Jeh.

During Taimur's time, I was psyched about having a normal delivery too. Then I had a crisis. It was my last scan, and I was a week away from delivery. Taimur was a big baby, and it turned out that the cord was around his neck. The sonologist called my ob-gyn and said they couldn't take a chance. I was so scared and really worried about my baby. Would he be okay? Then there was the disappointment. I had really wanted to have a normal delivery. In fact, I had never had a 'surgery' in my life. Who would willingly want a surgery?

But my doctor sat me down and explained to me that during labour, I would be pushing, the baby would be pulling, the cord was precarious. Anything could happen and it was better not to take a chance. Dr Feroze, Saif and I then took a joint decision. A nerve-wracking 48 hours later, I had Taimur via a C-section. I remember being wheeled in, being soothed by the nurse, hearing my anaesthesiologist's comforting words. Then everything was a blur.

I followed my doctor's orders; in fact, I followed all his advice through my pregnancy unquestioningly. Saif and I were very nervous. But I realized you just cannot control certain things. Jeh, by default, was a C baby too. If you've had one C, it is very hard to follow it up with a natural delivery. Most doctors advise against it. I waited till 40 weeks for Jeh and then opted for a C. I was very uncomfortable in the OT because Jeh was still very high and thus was pressing on my diaphragm. My back was intensely pressured too.

When Taimur was born, he didn't scream. The first thing Jeh did was scream! It resounded through the OT! Both my babies are so different. Tim looks a lot like Saif. Jeh looks like me. Taimur, however, is outgoing and flamboyant. I noticed that even when he was three months old. Jeh is a lot more intense, quieter.

Having Jeh during the pandemic meant my parents and sister couldn't visit me. Saif couldn't stay with me either. I spent three days in the hospital by myself, with all the nurses around me. Of course I felt alone. I would wear my N95 mask every time a nurse or doctor entered the room, which meant I was often nursing Jeh with a mask on. It was a strange feeling.

Post both births, I was adrift for the first seven days. It happens to all of us. I don't think I reacted very well to a Caesarean. The after-effects were also painful. Like any new mom, I was exhausted, I was lost. I don't think I slept. When Taimur was born, I don't think I even bathed every day! Both times, the scar and I took a while to heal.

With Taimur, I bled for a month. But with Jeh, I was bleeding even 60 days on. I did a postnatal sonography, in fact, to make sure everything was okay. Everything was indeed normal, but I guess my body just took a lot longer to get back. My feet were still swollen two months post delivery the second time around. My hormones were out of whack for a while. All the stuff people would say about your body taking a full six months to feel normal again – that didn't make sense to me before. But I felt it after I had Jeh. To put it simply, I felt awful.

Both times, when I felt especially low or tired, I would remind myself that this is what I always wanted in life. Eyes on the prize, as they say.

There was a day, shortly after I had Taimur, when I was alone in my room. I undressed for a shower. And I looked at myself in the mirror. Reality hit hard. There I was – scarred, chubby, puffy, tired. I saw the baby bulge, the dark circles, the dressing bandage of my C incision. I cannot describe how I felt. But then when I held Taimur in my arms, I felt like I could do this a million times over.

Within a few months of having Taimur, I felt upbeat again. I hit the gym in a little over a month. I was happy to go out. After having Jeh, I wouldn't say I was moody. But I was exhausted. Maybe it's because I had him at 40 or maybe it's because I am just so hands-on this time. I am doing things my way. I am setting his schedule and patterns and feeds. I am a lot more knowledgeable and confident. I grab him in my arms and walk up and down the stairs of my house all day with him. I don't remember feeling this adept when Taimur was a baby. I guess being locked down in the midst of a terrible Covid wave helped me bond with Jeh. There is no outing, no gym, no distraction. And second baby syndrome, I guess, right? You know what you're doing, and this second little fellow just grows up on his own.

Like all first-time moms, I was very anxious about breastfeeding. Would I lactate enough? Would my baby latch? In fact, I had worried about that through the pregnancy. I know a lot of moms take to it very easily and have enough breast milk supply. But I didn't have that luck. Taimur was an abrupt Caesarean. I literally had no milk for over 14 days. I was completely dry and I was a typical nervous first-time mom. He was given formula feeds from the first day.

God! What an awful time it was. I have vivid memories of those hazy days as I sat on a chair with Taimur in my arms, trying desperately to feed him. My mom and my nurse would be hovering by my side, pressing at my boobs and wondering why 'it' wasn't happening. Everyone gives you advice. You are under constant pressure. I wondered if there was something wrong with my body! Anyhow, I kept on and on trying (with medicines, satavari, gond, ghee – I did it all) and then managed to lactate a little.

I semi-nursed him for a few months thereafter and I even tried to express a little bit of milk occasionally. I used a lot of top feeds – he was hungry as hell, and I couldn't bear hearing him cry. I wasn't about to put my head to the floor and say I'm not lactating enough, so I should let my child go hungry! I did whatever I could.

With Jeh, I was definitely more relaxed because I knew the drill! I told myself from the beginning that I wouldn't beat myself up about breastfeeding. If it comes, it comes. But I had much better flow and did manage to nurse him. At night, I gave him some formula to top up his feed, if my feed wasn't enough for him or if I needed a couple of extra hours of sleep. Every day with him was different. Between last night to this morning, his appetite would go up an ounce! And, yes, I'll admit it – breastfeeding him (and doing it exclusively for a few weeks) felt like an achievement!

Look, there is a lot going on in your body and your mind. And there is no 'best mother' award coming to any of us. Every mother is a mother. It doesn't make you love your child any less. It doesn't make your child love you any less. I love my mom; I don't know if she breastfed me! I refuse to set any nursing goals for myself with Jeh. Such targets place too much pressure on you. Will I breastfeed for six months or one year? It all depends.

P.S.: During Taimur's time, I eventually made my peace with

my breastfeeding fears. But then just as I gave up one neurosis, I picked up a new stress about burping. I was totally neurotic about burping him! I don't know why! I would keep him on my shoulder for 20 minutes, refusing to put him down till I heard the burp. No matter how tiny it was. I had nightmares about him vomiting all the milk while he was sleeping. With Jeh, I knew better. But as a first-time mom – you don't know anything, and there is always going to be one worry or the other. It's the same with fathers too though, I guess. Saif, his past experience notwithstanding, was also as lost as me.

4

LABOUR AND CHILDBIRTH

My mom said I slipped out in 2.5 minutes while she was still making her way from the elevator to the room. There was no labour room and OT for me!

Your third trimester is pretty much a countdown to the finish line. There may be a lot of preparations you would have started even from trimester two: like prenatal classes (live, if available to you locally, or online), internationally accredited prenatal exercises, self-massages and labour research (Yes! It's happening soon!). The final sprint begins well before you reach your due date. As mentioned earlier, women deliver any time from 32 weeks up until 40 weeks – depending on whether it is a high-risk pregnancy, a complicated pregnancy, a singleton or multiple babies. A lot of moms derive great comfort from understanding the entire process of birthing well in advance, their pain relief options, a possible Caesarean, inducing labour and their immediately post-birth bodies and babies.

It's the first eight to ten days after birth that are particularly hard on any mother. This is when you are exhausted, lost and anxious. So let's look at this very last part of your pregnancy and the phase that follows immediately post childbirth, step by step.

How will I know I am in labour?

Labour happens in three stages. There are many women who don't realize they are in the first stage of labour. There are some who may spend a week in early labour or stage one of labour. There are some who end up at the hospital just in time to give birth! You may finish one or all phases of labour and then be rushed in to have a Caesarean. You may bypass all these stages completely if you have a predetermined Caesarean. There is no set rule for your body and your baby.

What are the pre-labour signs?

This phase can start a couple of weeks, a few days or a few hours before you actually go into labour. The symptoms are (you may feel some, all, or none of these): a sudden surge in energy before your due date, loose motions, a brown lumpy discharge in your underwear, signs of spotting, back pain or thigh pain. You might feel niggling menstrual cramp-like feelings – these are contractions in your uterus that are putting pressure on the cervix to start the dilation and effacement process. Many women are 1 cm dilated for even 8 to 10 days! As you inch closer to delivery, look out for signs of bleeding, your water breaking and your mucus plug passing.

What does actual labour feel like?

You'll know you've begun your labour when you start feeling regular contractions. Over time, your contractions will begin to get longer and become more intense while the time between each contraction gets shorter. These may be accompanied by your water breaking or your mucus plug being expelled (see section 'A glossary of labour terms'). Your initial contractions may not feel extremely painful – some women are not even aware that they are in labour until they hit active labour.

Here is what different women say about their varied experiences with labour pains:

1. It feels like waves of pain that radiate from the front to the back or vice versa. Or move from side to side.
2. This pain does not stop or ease with movement or a change of activity or position (the way it eases off during Braxton-Hicks).
3. It feels like you need to poop very badly, or as if you have severe menstrual cramp pains.
4. It can also feel like you have a huge and painful gas bubble or like a bowling ball (or elephant!) is pressing on your abdominal organs and your insides: essentially, you feel intense pressure.
4. Each contraction may feel like someone is vacuuming your organs downwards through your vagina.

What should I do?

Speak to your doctor right away. Unless the cramps (i.e., contractions) are suddenly too quick or too severe, you may be told to time your cramps before you actually head to the hospital. If you see a lot of blood and a big gush of amniotic fluid, rush to the hospital. If you have been practising Lamaze breathing (see Chapter 3: Your Third Trimester) – wait until the later part of your labour (as it intensifies) to start.

INDUCING LABOUR: WHAT DOES IT MEAN?

In 2018, the Indian College of Obstetricians & Gynaecologists (ICOG) and the Federation of Obstetric and Gynaecological Societies of India (FOGSI) compiled a roster of Good Clinical Practice Recommendations on the induction of labour. According to this dossier, a doctor-assisted induction of labour should only be performed if there are specific medical indications.

Essentially, your doctor has to weigh the pros of inducing labour versus continuing the pregnancy. And if an induction must happen, it should be in a monitored and equipped health facility (i.e., a hospital/nursing home which has provisions for a Caesarean delivery). Ideally, your doctor will wait for you to finish 39 weeks minimum before inducing labour.

Why would your doctor need to induce labour? Amongst the leading reasons are: (a) if you're very post-term, (b) you have placental, cervical or uterine issues, (c) foetal distress of any kind, (d) PPROM, hypertension, diabetes, twins, (e) stillbirth, (f) if your waters have broken, but there are no signs of labour. Labour will not be induced for a vaginal delivery, but if you have any medical issues, a breech baby, pelvis problems or infections, you will be wheeled in for a C-section right away.

What happens at this time? Your doctor will explain the need for medically assisted labour induction. You will need to provide informed and written consent for it. Based on the status of your cervical effacement, your doctor will use a vaginal pessary, an intracervical gel, a dose of oxytocin or (in non-urgent cases) Foley's catheter and a membrane sweep. Rely on your doctor to explain the process to you at this time. You and your baby will be monitored and evaluated closely for all parameters (both your heart rates, baby's position and weight, your blood pressure, etc.) before the induction of labour begins and continuously throughout the process.

If you're full term, you may be advised by well-meaning friends and family to try and induce your own labour process naturally. If you research this, you will find a variety of methods to start this process, like drinking castor oil, eating spicy foods, duck walking, stimulating your nipples, having sex, using herbs, exercising, consuming pineapples and papayas and so on. According to ICOG and FOGSI, none of these methods have any proven efficacy. In an ideal scenario, let your doctor stress about your being overdue, not you! Be gentle with yourself at this time.

Why would I end up with a Caesarean delivery?

Women across the world are psychologically primed to believe that a normal delivery is the real deal. We often have a rosy picture when it comes to the entire process of birthing naturally and vaginally. Many women report feeling guilty and depressed after undergoing a Caesarean, as it made them feel somewhat inadequate. But this is not how it is!

A C-section is defined as a surgery where a baby is delivered via a small incision made in the mother's lower abdomen (where the skin folds) and in her uterus. The Caesarean scar can eventually hide underneath your underwear for the rest of your life. A local anaesthetic numbs the body waist down for a Caesarean.

After the baby is retrieved, doctors remove the placenta either manually or wait for a spontaneous delivery. Like in a vaginal delivery, the baby is put on your body for a few seconds post birth. The paediatrician will follow the same protocol for your baby as for a vaginal birth. Your sutures will be completed and dressed before you leave for your room. You may fall asleep during this stage. In India, most C-sections are followed by complete 24-hour supine bed rest with a catheter inserted for urine.

Most women who have had healthy pregnancies aspire to a normal (i.e., vaginal) birth – unless something goes wrong. It is best to stay prepared by reading up and understanding why a C-section can happen.

- A breech or transverse baby
- Foetal distress in any form, including nuchal cord (when the umbilical cord is wrapped around the baby's neck) and meconium aspiration – when the baby has passed meconium in the amniotic fluid and is at risk of inhaling or consuming it
- Your baby's head is larger than your pelvic bone (cephalopelvic disproportion)
- Umbilical cord prolapse – when a portion of the cord comes out before the baby. The doctor checks the pulsation on the cord; if weak, you will need a Caesarean
- Total placenta previa; gestational diabetes; high blood pressure; infections; a fibroid or tumour in your uterus; placental abruption (separation) during the labour process
- Multiple babies; precious pregnancy; older mom
- Your labour gets arrested suddenly and doesn't resume after the doctor induces it
- Your body goes into stress and you are unable to deliver the baby

A planned or elective Caesarean is also very common if you have placental anomalies, breech baby, twins or a precious pregnancy. The only possible non-medical reason for a C-section is when it is requested by the mother specifically. This is a common practice in urban India too, though the trend is moving back to natural deliveries.

What are my options for pain relief during a vaginal birth?

Everyone has a different threshold of pain and endurance. Did you know that it is common for many moms to not be able to tolerate the pain they're going through and quit the process to opt for a Caesarean delivery? Explore the various pain relief options available to you in advance so you can be prepared. Many women choose to birth without the use of pain relief too – it is entirely your choice.

- **Epidural**: This is the most widely used method of pain relief during childbirth. It is a local anaesthetic injected into your 'epidural' space in the spinal cord. Your attending anaesthesiologist will numb the spot on your lower back where the epidural is administered. You will then be awake and alert but numb from the belly down. Can it fail? Yes, rarely, but it happens. Advantages: Your pain is muted. Disadvantages: You may not feel the full strength of your contractions and will have to rely on your doctor and nurse to tell you when to push. On an average, it is ideal to opt for an epidural when you have dilated 4 to 5 cm or more. It takes 15–20 minutes to place the epidural catheter into your lower back and for the effect to kick in. Don't worry, no one expects you to know how dilated you are! Let your doctor know well in advance that you'd like an epidural during childbirth, so they're prepared to administer it at the right time. When you're near fully dilated (see section 'I've never done this before! Navigating the labour process') – it is too late for an epidural. Your doctor will tell you as much.

- **TENS machine**: The TENS machine (i.e., Transcutaneous Electrical Nerve Stimulation) is a small device used in physiotherapy that sends low voltage electrical currents to your body through flat electrodes (not needles) that can be stuck to your skin. You can stick these electrodes to your back. The electrical impulses block the pain signals sent to your brain. If you're in for high-tech, pick up this machine in advance and figure out how things work. You can find and buy a TENS machine online. It is used by women to help ease lower back pain during the **early** stages of labour (it has not proven to be very effective during the later stages of labour when contractions get stronger and more frequent). Since the risk to foetal development is still unknown, it is **not** safe to use a TENS machine until you have crossed 37 weeks of pregnancy.

- **Nitrous oxide**: Yes, that's right. Good old laughing gas. You can choose to start or stop nitrous oxide at any time during labour. You breathe it in through a mask. You can walk around while using it. Does it actually numb your pain? Nitrous oxide slows down your nervous system and makes you feel calm and content (and possibly giggly). For many women who are too late into their labour to exercise the epidural option, laughing gas can be a fallback. Your anaesthesiologist will make you breathe it in just as a contraction begins. Women who choose water birth can use nitrous oxide in the birthing pool.

A glossary of labour terms

Mucus plug: It is a sticky, gel-like secretion from your cervix that is expelled with a bit of blood during the early phase of labour. At the risk of sounding macabre, it is also called 'bloody show'. Losing your mucus plug does not hurt.

Water breaking: This is the breaking of your amniotic sac. It could be a gush, like it happens in movies. But this happens literally to fewer than 10 per cent of women. For most others, it is a trickle/leak – you might be sitting on the toilet and not even realize your water broke. You'll assume you're peeing. Waters can also break twice. Your water breaking is a sign that you will be in active labour effective immediately or in 24 hours or so. Only a small percentage of women report that their water broke much before they entered their active stage of labour. Some women also go into labour before their water breaks. In this case, your doctor will break your amniotic sac. This is called an amniotomy. If your cervix is dilated enough, your doctor will insert a slim, hooked instrument through your vagina and gently break your sac to let the fluid flow from your uterus into the cervix and out. Does it hurt? Well, no more than any vaginal/endo-pelvic exam.

Dilate/Dilated/Dilation: As you know, your cervix is the 3- to 4-cm-long muscle that connects your uterus with your vagina. It remains closed during your pregnancy to protect your baby and your body from infections. When your contractions first begin, it means the muscles in the walls of your uterus are starting their work. The contractions place pressure on your cervix, and it begins to open up slowly. As your cervix opens up, your ob-gyn will address it as 'dilation' and measure it in centimetre. It goes from 1 cm (i.e., a Cheerio or a blueberry) till 10 cm (i.e., a small cantaloupe, a bagel or, well, a baby's head). Your doctor will measure your dilation to check how far along into labour you are.

Effacement: This is the gradual thinning, shortening and drawing up of the cervix that happens during the process of labour. It will be measured in percentage from 0 to 100 per cent. Dilation and effacement go hand in hand as your labour progresses.

Nonstress Test (NST): It is a simple, non-invasive and risk-free 20- to 40-minute method to check on your baby's health during trimester three; if you're a high-risk mother, if you're overdue, if you're in labour or if your doctor or you have any concerns about the well-being of your baby. It is a simple foetal monitor that is placed over your bump. The NST checks if the baby is getting enough oxygen, her heartbeat, her movements and your contractions. The NST will reveal if you need further tests or if you're ready for delivery. The NST result will be reactive (baby's heart rate increases) or non-reactive (baby's heart rate does not increase and baby does not move in 60–90 minutes).

What happens during your labour

It's understandable that you're nervous. The actual act of birthing your baby is probably amongst the most daunting aspects of your entire pregnancy. So let's try and break down the process of labour in detail: what to expect, how to track your labour, what happens at the hospital and how you may feel until the baby finally arrives.

While most women choose the father of their child to be their birthing partner, there are some who will also choose their mother, friend, relative or a paid doula. It is entirely up to you. It is highly likely that only one person can enter the hospital with you and stay till you're discharged. Bear that in mind as you and your birthing partner prepare for the hospital.

I. Stage one

Stage one begins at your first hint of steady contractions (which you may or may not feel) and ends when you are ready to deliver your baby, i.e., essentially from the time you are 1 cm dilated till 10 cm. There is no fixed timeline for how long stage one of labour can last. It can go on for 18–20 hours for first-timers, while subsequent pregnancies could go up to six hours or so.

What is this discomfort that you feel? In the first stage of labour, it is your uterine contraction and dilation. In the second stage, it comes from your stretching birth canal, perineum and vulva.

In stage one, there is an **early phase**. Your body can display signs of early labour a few weeks or a few hours before you're ready to give birth. Here is the checklist for you to observe:

- A change in your bowel movement
- Contractions are irregular, mild, infrequent, bearable
- Changes in vaginal discharge
- Loss of appetite
- Joints feel looser
- Water break/leak
- Nesting instinct kicking in
- Bloody show (when the mucus plug discharges)
- A shift in your belly position (the baby drops)

Many women can have early labour symptoms for even 8 to 10 days. During this time, you can stay at home or continue to be active. You needn't rush to the hospital.

When your contractions occur 15–20 minutes apart and last 50–60 seconds each time, you leave for the hospital. This stage can last for several hours – till you are dilated 10 cm, and the baby is ready to birth.

What happens at the hospital? When you reach the hospital, you will check in with your paperwork. You may be given a room or sent straight to the labour room. The labour room will look a little bit like your regular hospital room, except perhaps bigger. It doesn't really have any equipment for you or your baby; so this isn't where you will be birthing your baby.

The nurses will monitor your blood pressure. Depending on the directive of your doctor, the nurses *may* give you an enema (to clear your system), may shave your pubic hair and hook you up to an NST machine. (In case you're wondering, your pubic hair can be shaved for a vaginal birth and even for a Caesarean for visibility during the birth process and for the sutures that come later.) The NST is not mandatory; you can also be examined physically with a foetoscope.

You can consider your pain relief options at this stage, based on how dilated you are. The doctor or nurse attending to you will be keeping track.

If you're able to, walk around. Breathe through your contractions on your fours or stand and lean forward (on to a wall or your partner). You will probably be pacing around alone with your partner at this point. Many moms try squats and duck walks. You can sit back on your ankles with your belly sinking to your knees and try and lean forward with lots of pillow support.

Most hospitals in India tend to put you down on your back.

Fight the urge and find a way to be more mobile to relieve your back pain and discomfort. The nurse will come and go to keep an eye on you. You may feel a terrible urge to poop as each contraction comes. But it is the pressure on your uterus. Your doctor may also pop around to give you a little word of confidence and check on your progress. If you feel like you need some rest, try and get some sleep. There are moms who report taking a catnap at some point of time during the prolonged phase of early labour.

How can your partner help?

Encourage her to stay relaxed at home in the early stages of labour, until the time is right to head to the hospital. During stage one, walk with her. Encourage her to change positions. A relaxing, kneading massage on the lower back as she lies on her side or leans forward may really help. Hold her hand and help her focus on breathing through the contractions. Wear comfortable clothes and carry something warm for yourself, in case you end up spending hours on a cold hospital floor. Play some soothing music if you feel it may calm her down.

The **active phase** is a part of stage one of labour. The cervix is about 4 cm dilated by now. The contractions become regular, more intense, more frequent and uncomfortable. **Now, contractions occur five minutes apart and last 50–60 seconds, and then three minutes apart and last 45 seconds.** You will feel intense pressure in your lower back and rectum. Your mucus plug and amniotic fluid will likely pass. If your waters don't break naturally, your doctor will usually wait for about 70 per cent of this phase to pass before choosing to manually rupture your amniotic sac. This is a physically intense stage. You may have slipped into a serious and quiet mode, while many other moms say they were screaming at their spouses and throwing things! This active stage may last four to eight hours or more.

Your blood pressure, pulse and temperature will be monitored. Your doctor/nurse will do a quick pelvic exam and check the dilation and effacement. You will likely have been changed into a hospital gown, if you haven't been changed already. Don't fret if you find yourself getting irritable as the exhaustion and waves of pain wear you down. A lot of moms say they go in with the intention of being poised, elegant and in control, but – really – you can never tell where this is going to go.

Try and use the time between contractions to walk around. Keep urinating. Keep up with the breathing. It's only a matter of time now! The baby is nearly here.

Your contractions will now go to two to three minutes apart and last for 60 seconds. You could be going nuts by now. Many moms have found nibbling on ice chips helpful at this stage. Walk around – but only if you're up for it. You may go from feeling hot to cold. You may feel like giving up.

Your legs may tremble, and your body may shake – it's the hormones prepping for birth. This is the time for Lamaze breathing or just regular, controlled, deep relaxing breaths – remember you will be fighting the urge to push. You cannot push until your doctor gives you the go-ahead. This active stage ends when you are 10 cm dilated. You'll be headed to the OT now.

How can your partner help?

Do not let her push until the doctor gives the go-ahead. Keep telling her she is doing well! Hold her hand. Between pushes, remind her to rest. She may feel like throwing up at this stage, so keep a cold towel handy. The birthing stage is generally a high pressure one. Stay positive and encourage her to breathe. Your reassurance and the soothing words of the supporting doctors and nurses are what will tide her through this intense period.

II. Stage two

This is when you will give birth to your baby. Your ob-gyn will attend to you with their full attention now. If you need an episiotomy, you will be given a local anaesthetic before your doctor makes the cut. An intravenous (IV) drip is standard protocol during childbirth. Here, a needle will be inserted into a vein (most commonly on the back of your hand). A cannula is pushed over the needle and taped up to keep it in place. The cannula remains in your hand. The attached IV bag will then transfer the required medication into your bloodstream (painkillers, antibiotics and so on) as needed through the cannula. Your doctor may sometimes choose to retain the cannula on your hand for 24 to 48 hours post birth, just in case any medicines need to be administered suddenly.

This sounds like a lot when you're reading it here – but all of it will be a whirlwind of activity. You will be prepped for birth in a matter of minutes. When you are 10 cm dilated, your doctor will give you the go-ahead to push after your next contraction. Some moms feel a pang of embarrassment – that their legs are splayed open and their bodies are on display. Yes, you are vulnerable in these moments. You know most women end up passing stool on the table? You may hear the nurse saying it. Someone may lunge to clean it up. It may feel like the most embarrassing moment of your life. But you have to relinquish control for this duration of time. It will be over soon!

Now, the contractions will slow down to two to three minutes apart and go on for 90 seconds. You will be asked to hold your breath in and then push while breathing out slowly. Remember when you push, curl your body forward. And you want to know what this push really is? Like you are constipated and are trying very hard to poop! Some doctors describe it as a 'potty push'. This is the basic momentum of your pushing. There – now you know what you're in for!

Across the world, women squat, stand, rest on their hands and knees or lie on their side with one leg up during the process of pushing. Indian hospitals are generally focused on lying on the back propped up. Pushing in a squatting position is encouraged too. Addressing birthing positions with your doctor in advance might help.

WHAT IS A FORCEPS OR VACUUM-ASSISTED VAGINAL BIRTH?

There are two indications for a forceps or vacuum-assisted birth. The first is to reduce the length of the second phase of labour because the mother has heart disease or other issues (like maternal exhaustion, high BP, a vaginal delivery after a previous C-section) and cannot bear the prolonged pushing period. The second is when the baby shows signs of distress or meconium stained liquor (MSL) while coming down the birthing passage. Here, the delivery is expedited using one of these means so that the baby can be attended to as quickly as possible by the attending paediatrician. Do note that if you have a large baby or if your baby's head or body is too large and the shoulder gets stuck in the birth canal – i.e., shoulder dystocia – both are actually contraindications to the application of forceps or vacuum.

There is no fixed answer for the process of birthing. Typically, this phase can go on for about two hours. The toughest part is the baby's head and one shoulder emerging; after that it is much smoother. In a few seconds you'll know if it's a boy or a girl.

Many women say stage two of labour was a haze of memories. The entire support staff in the OT is singing out your name – encouraging you to push. Your doctor, of course, is instructing you every step of the way. If you're amped up on an epidural, you may be numbed against the active pain, but you will be using your doctor's cues on when to push. The baby birthing teams at most hospitals function as a pretty cohesive unit; they're attuned to each other and can read each other's eye signals and body language! They're vigilant about you and your baby. So allow yourself to be guided by your attending doctors.

It feels surreal at this point. Like you're the star of a show and everyone's chanting your name! A lot of moms say they allowed themselves to channel this support; take strength from it. And, from this haze, what they do remember is a tiny creature being placed on their bare skin – quite suddenly. For a few short seconds. And then taken away. Your baby has arrived. This 'skin-to-skin' contact, also called kangaroo care, is now a standard practice at birth. Your paediatrician will place your naked baby on your bare abdomen immediately post birth, before taking her away to check her out.

Your ob-gyn will carefully clamp the umbilical cord in two places and cut it. Delayed clamping of the cord is now standard practice across hospitals (see box 'What is DCC?'). The baby is then handed over to the paediatrician who, with a battery of nurses, is cleaning, weighing, measuring and caring for your baby. You may not be able to see all this at the moment. But a lot is happening.

WHAT IS DCC?

Delayed cord clamping (DCC) is basically when all your attending doctors prolong the time between the delivery of the baby and the cutting of the umbilical cord. The time varies from 30 seconds till 3 to 5 minutes or after the placenta is delivered and till the time the cord stops pulsating. Typically, the cord pulsates till roughly 5 minutes post birth. The advantages are that the cord blood continues to be transferred into your baby even after she is born. This is very important. If you've opted for cord blood banking, it would be best to discuss the pros and cons with your paediatrician in advance.

III. Stage three

This 'afterbirth' stage lasts a few minutes (going up to about 20 minutes) while your body expels the placenta. After this, your uterus still continues to contract, but this will be mild (like a period cramp) and may continue for a few days. As soon as you give birth, a little of the cord blood will be taken to identify your baby's blood group and process some basic reports (like thyroid and G6PD). In case you've opted for cord blood collection, this is when it will happen. The Apgar assessment of your baby is done by the attending paediatrician. Your baby will be cleaned up and dried. Your baby's nasal and mouth passages will be suctioned gently if required – this is especially the case with Caesarean babies because they come straight out of water. If your baby's eyes are sticky, the paediatrician will put eye drops. This happens more during vaginal deliveries when vaginal contamination gets into the baby's eyes. A vitamin K injection is given soon to the baby after birth, a default practice all over the world. This is because vitamin K plays an important role in preventing haemorrhaging. Your paediatrician may also gently pass catheters through till your baby's abdomen to check for blockages and another at the anus to check if it is patent.

When your baby is handed over to you again, you will see her properly for the first time. A warm fuzzy bundle, wrapped in a standard-issue hospital swaddle, will be placed across your chest. This is when your paediatrician may encourage you to try and suckle her, even if it is for a couple of minutes. This is simply to encourage the reflex of lactation. Your baby may not be able to do anything right now – it's okay. If you find her in the mood to suckle, ask a nurse for help with the latching. When she is given to you, you will see she is breathing heavily – her little nostrils flaring and settling. Your baby is reeling from her journey out into the world just as much as you're reeling from the process of birthing her.

Your heart will melt through the discomfort, the emotions and the tears. That's it! You're a mom!

You and your baby will receive identical identifying wristbands (it might also be placed on your baby's ankle, depending on the hospital policy). This will be checked every time your baby is taken in and out of your presence, and it must come off only when you exit the hospital. As per protocol in Indian hospitals, babies are wheeled into the nursery shortly after birth, while your ob-gyn tends to you. Your doctor will examine your placenta to make sure it has come out as a whole and then stitch you up as needed. Your baby will be kept in a warmer for 30 minutes post birth. She will be transferred into your room pretty much as soon as you are. You must make sure this happens. This is called 'rooming in'.

Do you remember when you rode your last roller coaster? You get in the train, buckle up and push off slowly. That is when you first figure you are pregnant. Then you're riding that steep uphill track, chugging away. The anticipation of what's to come is already killing you! That's your 40 weeks in a nutshell. And childbirth? Well, rushing down the track full throttle and doing a series of flips, turns and loop-the-loops until you finally slow down and screech to a halt.

You may slip into a deep sleep at this point – it is the anaesthetic, the relief, the exhaustion. Congratulations! It's done.

Understanding an episiotomy vs natural tearing

Natural tearing is precisely that – when your vagina tears naturally in the process of childbirth. On the other hand, before you give birth vaginally, your doctor may make a surgical incision – an episiotomy cut – at the opening of your vagina to make it bigger. This is in the perineum area – i.e., the tissue between the vagina and anus. A quick local anaesthetic is administered before the doctor makes the cut. It is sutured post delivery.

The debate on what is better between an episiotomy and natural tearing has been an ongoing one. Why? During the birth process, natural tears can go from the perineum's skin to the muscles and extend to the rectum (sometimes, they can extend upwards and damage the urethra). These are called third and fourth degree tears. Some medical practitioners stand by the better recovery process of natural tears though.

However, some doctors prefer a pre-planned episiotomy to avoid natural tearing of the tissue and maintain control of the birthing process. An episiotomy cut is made to avoid third or fourth degree perineal tears, especially if the baby's head size is large, the baby is in the occipito-posterior position (i.e., looking towards the mother's front) or when forceps or vacuum is to be applied. But there are times when an episiotomy also results in further third and fourth degree natural tearing of the perineum, till the anus. The healing process post both these options depends on the degree of tearing.

The American College of Obstetricians and Gynecologists

(ACOG) made a recommendation in 2006 against the routine use of episiotomies. In India, while the precise numbers are uncertain, it is a part of most vaginal deliveries (up to 77 per cent), especially at private hospitals. You can discuss this ahead of time with your doctor.

Alternative birthing

As we discussed in **Part I: Your 40 Weeks**, if you're considering the assistance of a doula or a hypnobirthing practitioner or even a water birth, your research should be complete before trimester three. Why? Because trimester three is the execution phase! Any tool of alternative birthing may also alter the outcome of your childbirth process. Let's take a deep dive into the three tools of alternative birthing options available in India and understand what each one means.

Who is a doula?

With Sanam M. Manchanda, CLD, CLE, CCE (USA), internationally certified labour doula, childbirth and lactation educator, newborn massage practitioner; www.newbeginningz.in

The concept of a doula is centuries old. It's just that the word 'doula' has come to us from the West. A doula has no formal medical experience. She supports the mom-to-be or the parents-to-be for a positive and natural birthing experience. A doula does not replace your obstetrician/gynaecologist.

A pregnant woman can approach and enlist the services of

a doula in advance. Moms choose to book a doula any time from their first trimester till the last few days before delivery. A doula can then assist you from the start of your labour process (while you're still at home) until you give birth. There are some doulas who are qualified to assist you through your prenatal preparations and your pregnancy milestones followed by labour, childbirth and postpartum care too, like baby massages, lactation consultations and self-care.

However, if you're giving birth at a private or public hospital or a nursing home, you will need to take the hospital policies into account. Although still uncommon, women opting for a doula-assisted birth have increased in the past 10 years. A doula's role depends on how supportive your hospital and your doctor are. Depending on the protocol that your medical centre and practitioners follow, a doula and your birthing partner may both not be present with you during childbirth. You may have to pick just one person to be with you. You will have to check with your hospital.

Now, what does a doula do while you're in labour? She will be your mother or your best friend! She assists a labouring mom by helping her use birthing positions favoured by gravity (like squatting, birth balls or standing and so on). She will stay with you every second, no matter how long your labour lasts, helping you breathe correctly and relax. She knows what massage will make you feel better in your final stages of labour, she can read your cues and help you stay calm. Her words and directives will be firm and comforting. A doula also ensures that the first few minutes of skin-to-skin contact between your newborn baby and you can take place and will encourage you to attempt your first round of breastfeeding at the earliest.

What is water birthing?

With Dr Ameet Dhurandar, obstetrician and gynaecologist (MDDGO) and trained water birthing and hypnobirthing practitioner; www.waterbirthmumbai.com

Water birthing relies heavily on the premise of gentle vaginal birthing – with minimal medical intervention (no epidural, oxytocin or pitocin), no screaming, no noises! It is still an unconventional approach to birthing in India. There are a select few water birthing centres (or hospitals that are enabled with water birthing pools) across some big cities in India. Most centres see about three to four (or less) successful water births in a month. The primary requirement is that the mom is physically fit and mentally strong. Age doesn't matter. But maternal distress (like high blood pressure), a big baby, placental/cervical complications, IUGR or fever are definite contraindications. High-risk pregnancies are not ideal for water birthing.

What is the key to this process? That the birthing mom must relax. And water is a great tool for relaxation. When you relax, your endorphins kick in. The basis of natural water birthing is that women are designed to birth on their own. The birthing mom spends her time with meditation, breathing, music, birthing balls, squats, hypnobirthing and staying hydrated. Your doctor is always available to step in and help if there is a problem, although the doctor is officially meant to step in only at the later stage of active labour. You will deliver with a doctor at your side. Many water birth practitioners in India encourage you to enlist the services of a doula.

When you're about 6 to 7 cm dilated, you will be led into the pool. The lights are dim; everything quiet and free of stimulus.

Your partner can enter the pool with you. You should deliver within about two hours of easing into the pool. If there is no progress, your situation is reassessed. If your body or your baby go into stress, the situation is reassessed again. There are moms who start off with the intention of having a natural vaginal water birth, but seek medical intervention or painkillers in between. After all, this is a natural process and, ultimately, things can go their own way.

A lot of moms may wonder if their babies could drown in water. They can't! Remember, it takes them time to gasp for their first breath of air and to pink up. Your baby is coming from fluid (amniotic sac) into fluid (the pool)! Your water birthing doctor will be particular about skin-to-skin contact and immediate suckling (even if your birth process ends up in a Caesarean). The nipple stimulation produces hormones to eject the placenta naturally. If you would like to consider a water birth, look for a centre with an NICU and paediatricians on call. The risks of an infection occurring are the same as with any other delivery choice.

Can hypnobirthing ensure a pain-free delivery?

With Kritika Khona, hypnobirthing practitioner, hypnotherapist (CHt), psychotherapist, NLP practitioner and remedial educator

Essentially, this is a regular practice of hypnosis, positive visualization and intense relaxation techniques that are used by a pregnant woman (and her partner) to relax her body and assuage her fears of labour and childbirth. A lot of women wonder if using hypnobirthing is a pain-free experience or a medication-free one. Actually, using the techniques of hypnobirthing means you achieve a deep state of relaxation for your mind and body, which enables you to focus on birthing, rather than on the pain or discomfort. Of course, every woman feels birthing pain in surges, but you can respond to these surges in a healthy manner and go on to birth calmly and smoothly. Hypnobirthing is still a fairly uncommonly used tool for childbirth, although there are now more hypnobirthing practitioners in bigger cities like Mumbai and Delhi. If you research hypnobirthing online you will find studies that have implications on the length and intensity of labour, reduced rates of medical intervention and pain relief medication and also improved outcomes on postpartum depression. A hypnobirth practitioner will not necessarily assist you through your birthing process, like a doula can. Instead, most often, a practitioner will train the mom-to-be and her partner through a series of hypnobirthing sessions before the end of term, in order to equip them with the necessary skills to handle childbirth.

5

YOUR FIRST TWO WEEKS AFTER DELIVERY

Whether it's a Caesarean or a vaginal birth, you may fall asleep after you've said your first hello to your baby and while the doctor is still suturing you. A lot of mums are wired too – awake, chatting and excited about this new little being. When your doctor is done with you, you'll be wheeled into your room. This is usually a moment of great fanfare – your waiting family members grinning and waving at you in excitement, maybe a few high-fives along the way!

What happens to you in the first few hours post the birth of your baby?

You might wake up to find yourself in a quiet room. Your baby may already be in there with you, on a cot placed next to your bed. You may feel absolutely fine – hungry as a horse and raring to go. But there is a good chance you could also be groggy, sore and exhausted.

Many women report feeling bouts of extreme chills, a tingling or pins and needles on their hands and feet, uncontrollable shaking, hand tremors and severe itching across the body. Don't worry! It's a reaction of your body to the stress of childbirth, to the anaesthetic which is wearing off by now, the sudden retreat of those crazy hormones and, also, severe exhaustion. Report these symptoms immediately to your doctor and ask for a consultation. Something like an itch, for instance, can be fixed with an antihistamine injection. A change of antibiotic/painkiller may also help you relax. The cannula that may still be inserted in the back of your hand for the IV drip may cause a little discomfort, itching or swelling beyond the first day or so. If the swelling becomes very bothersome, speak to your nurse or doctor about switching hands. Use a medicated topical ointment for the hand swelling (thrombosis).

Now, breastfeeding! Speak to your paediatrician in advance about this, if you have a chance. Else, ask your doctor, a lactation consultant or friends and family members who have had babies recently. When should you begin to breastfeed? Within the first hour or first few hours post birth, if you can! Ask for your baby to be given to you early on, if this hasn't already happened for any reason. In case your baby needs to remain in the NICU for any reason, you could use a breast pump and start pumping. This early suckling (or pumping) encourages the lactation reflex to kick in.

Lactation experts will encourage you to: (a) let your baby feel your skin, (b) keep him awake while nursing, (c) begin to master the full areola latch from day one (a nipple latch will cause soreness in no time and make you feel like hell every time you nurse. The milk ducts are around the areola and not on the nipple). On an average, it could take 24 to 48 hours or more for your breast to be filled with milk. So be patient with yourself. Milk is activated with a reflex (called 'let down'), and this reflex needs a stimulus: hence the attempt to breastfeed soon after birth.

Depending on your doctor's protocol and the extent of your suturing, you might be heavily medicated with painkillers and antibiotics. You may even be 'nil-by-mouth', which means you won't be consuming anything except a few spoons of water. With a Caesarean, you may be on complete bed rest for 24 hours. Your incision and your insides may hurt in waves – ask for a painkiller suppository as these are very effective (bear in mind that a C is a full-blown surgery!). Be prepared for some tough love post a C. Your doctor is quite likely to get you to start moving in 24 hours.

Your vaginal birth sutures may also feel stingy and itchy. Your nurses will be putting ointment on you. The nurses will be helping you change your blood-soiled pads too. The best advice seasoned moms can give is this: surrender! You will be tended to like a child. There are no filters. Rest assured, after this you are unlikely to feel self-conscious when getting a massage buck naked – forever!

You will bleed for anything from 10 days to six weeks post the delivery. What is this postpartum bleeding about? This vaginal bleeding and discharge (termed as lochia) is all the extra blood and tissue from your uterus that's done its job for nine months. It starts as bright red, with occasional lumps. It is heavy at first and then peters out. You may bleed less while you're resting and more (even gushing) when you walk around. Remember, it is ideal to use a good quality sanitary napkin till your postpartum bleeding stops – not a tampon. Doctors also recommend you use a non-synthetic sanitary pad for the first few days.

If the bleeding is very heavy, foul smelling and accompanied by pain and fever, call your doctor. It could be an infection of the uterus. Please note that a very heavy bleed, called postpartum haemorrhage, can cause a very serious drop in blood pressure and can be dangerous. It can happen in the first 24 hours or even 12 weeks post delivery. You may see big clots and a lot of blood and feel cold, nauseous, dizzy or weak. It can happen because of issues in the uterus, vagina or cervix, or due to twin births, prolonged labour, high blood pressure, a reaction to the anaesthetic and so on.

COMPLICATIONS: POST-BIRTH PROBLEMS

A pelvic organ prolapse is a type of hernia. It occurs when the pelvic muscles weaken and cause pelvic organs – like the bladder, uterus, rectum – to 'fall' (or 'prolapse') into the vagina. While a mild case can improve on its own, some cases may require surgery. It is not a very commonly occurring issue. You will feel a downward pressure in your vagina, like something is falling out of it, or like you're sitting on a ball. A vaginal prolapse falls into the same category and can be described as a condition when your anterior or posterior vaginal wall prolapses. Again, either pelvic strengthening exercises or surgery may work. Additionally, some women complain of diastasis recti, which is when your abdominal muscles separate as your belly grows and protrude slightly. In this case, you will feel bumps and soreness around your belly for months post birth. The solution? Seriously well-targeted core strengthening exercises (see Chapter 9: Fitness).

A look at the first eight to ten days post birth

Your time in the hospital

You will be in the hospital for about two to three days if you have had a normal delivery without complications and typically three to five days if you have had a C-section.

Your baby's paediatric exam will happen within 24 hours post birth and every day thereafter while you're in the hospital. The paediatrician will ask about your baby's urine, stool and reflux to slowly assess his well-being. A hearing test is important. A small, delicate instrument is used on your baby when he is quiet. It checks the hearing accurately, post day two or three of birth. You may also get a 'deferred' reading. Don't panic. Your doctor will repeat the hearing test after two weeks. As any paediatrician will tell you, a new mom will find any reason to cry! Over the next few weeks, you're fragile and overwrought – even stray remarks can pull you down. So, do be kind to yourself.

You will be asked for permission for the neonatal metabolic screening programme for your baby, where about four drops of blood will be collected from your baby in the first 48 hours and screened for metabolic anomalies. Do make sure you opt for this test. These reports take 10 days to process. In case there are anomalies, your doctor/hospital will quite likely repeat this test to be sure, and you will be asked for another sample. If your baby does have any metabolic disorders, remember these are inherent. A change of diet, lifestyle and medication from an early stage can really keep your child stable.

Your baby's BCG and Hepatitis B vaccines and OPV (oral polio vaccine) will also happen within the first 24 hours post birth. Your next round of baby vaccines will happen 30 to 45 days post birth. A month post birth is also the time around which your ob-gyn will call you in for a post-delivery check-up.

Whether it is a normal vaginal birth or a C-section, get moving as soon as your doctor gives you the go-ahead in the hospital room. In a normal vaginal birth, you may just be up and about on the same day. With a C-section, this may happen 24 hours later. Your doctor and nurses will encourage you to use the bathroom by yourself so you start to gain confidence. If you have had an episiotomy or tears during a vaginal birth, you will have a few stitches in your perineum. Your doctor may encourage you to sit in a warm sitz bath in your hospital bathroom and then continue it at home. A doughnut shaped air cushion will really help you to sit comfortably. Remember, it is ideal to keep your stitches clean and dry. You will be asked to use an ointment on your stitches for several days.

If you're in discomfort, you could go ahead and ask for a painkiller to take either orally or as a suppository. Women are given a laxative post birth, so their stool passes easily and without pressure. Continue to use that laxative as per your doctor's prescription. A lot of women find themselves dealing with an inordinate fear of passing their first stool. If you've had a vaginal birth especially, you may literally fear that your stitches will burst open. But don't worry, this is not going to happen.

Stick to cotton underwear and comfortable pants – it helps in both cases, a vaginal birth and a C. Post a C-section, chances are you will be supine in bed with a catheter for urine for at the least one whole day. Your stitches will take a while to heal. Use a cushion or a pillow on your stitches, if you need to laugh or sneeze! Take help to get in and out of bed. Some women do indeed find it harder to recover post a C than others. There is no fixed rule for the way a body reacts to a surgery.

Coming home

The first day that you're home, you will most likely be dazed. There is a new human who is dependent on you, and the sense of responsibility can crash upon you like a real tsunami. Most first-time parents feel overwhelmed returning home and especially when they are finally left alone with their little baby. What do we do next, they wonder in panic!

But this is when you breathe. All the knowledge you've gathered through your nine months, the prenatal classes you may have done, the physical and mental preparations for your baby, and the doctors, friends and family you may have spoken to – this will hold you in good stead.

These first eight to ten days are the key to observing your baby and gauging his well-being. Like, is he suckling eagerly after a four-hour break (breast or bottle)? Or, is he passing enough urine; your four-day-old baby should at the least be peeing four times a day. In the early stages, your baby will pass loose and watery stool, maybe even frequently. It is normal and it is not called diarrhoea. It is usually post the 15-day baby check-up that your paediatrician will breathe easy, as will you.

What are the worries that consume most mothers immediately post delivery? Well, at the top of the list is – you guessed it – breastfeeding. Breast milk is considered the best food for your baby, wholesome and immunizing. It's also the most sterile and fuss-free way to feed your baby. The American Academy of Paediatrics recommends that mothers breastfeed for 12 months, and the WHO says babies should be exclusively breastfed for six months (i.e., without solids and liquids, not even water).

Yes, breastfeeding is an innate reflex, and many moms feel

a sense of complete bliss when they're alone with their baby, nursing the little one. But while it comes easily to so many women, there are still others who may find it difficult to nurse their babies, and the guilt that comes with this can be crushing (see section 'Help! I can't breastfeed'). In fact, studies abroad point to the fact that most moms around the world don't manage to exclusively breastfeed their children till the WHO guideline of six months. A tip that will come in handy through those long days and nights of breastfeeding is to always resist the urge to 'comfort-feed' your baby. Many moms bring their babies to their breast at the slightest hint of unrest, and spending hours and hours with a baby at your breast can be exhausting and stressful.

Now, the other big thing. Many moms will go through baby blues, postpartum anxiety (PPA) or postpartum depression (PPD), which may vary from mild to severe. Many experts prefer to define these mood disorders under the umbrella of 'peripartum depression'. Essentially, the state of hormonal, physiological, biological and emotional flux can commence at *any* point of time during a pregnancy and then linger on for longer.

India reports about one crore cases of pregnancy mood disorders of various types. According to a WHO review and analysis on postpartum depression in India in 2017, about 22 per cent Indian mothers report having postpartum depression. The global prevalence stands at about 10 per cent of births. However, the degrees vary.

PPA usually resolves in a few weeks and might require only reassurance and counselling. More severe is PPD. Women with a previous history of depression or a severely stressful past event are even more susceptible. These feelings can come on without warning. Your hormones are getting back to their pre-pregnancy state, and there are multiple changes to your life and body. You may have bouts of irritability, mood swings, demands and tears. Other moms might have a more intense version of this – showing loss of appetite, sadness, disinterest, low energy, difficulty sleeping, difficulty bonding with the baby, fear that they're not good moms, inability to think clearly, thoughts of self-harm and feelings of shame or inadequacy.

Depression and anxiety disorders are not uncommon at these times and might be more pronounced after childbirth. Please don't shy away from seeking medical advice about your troubles. Not all of this is in your control! It's a genuine and common medical condition, and you will require help for it. If you have a great social support system, you can work through this with the help of your partner, parents, friends, family, a psychiatrist or even a counsellor. The best thing would be to first speak to your ob-gyn. Many Indian women land up remaining undiagnosed. And the complications could be the start of a chronic depressive illness (see section 'Peripartum depression with Dr Prabha Chandra').

One of the other big sensations of the first ten days (indeed the early months) is going to be exhaustion. Your baby will need to be fed every three hours, and you may feel you are sleepwalking through the days. Ensure you have help especially in the night feeds. This is a great time for your partner to swoop in and share the load. Your partner/family member can do the grunt work of picking the baby up, bringing him to you and burping him after the feed. Some of you might have a nanny to help in the night, if you can afford one. Yet be warned, despite the support, you are going to feel more tired than you have ever felt.

Many moms also find it painful to confront their post-delivery body in the early days. If you look into a mirror, you'll see a bumped, bruised, sore body. You'll see disproportionately large breasts. Your nipples may be chafed. (Here's a quick tip: After you feed your baby, squeeze out a few drops of breast milk, brush it on to your areolas and let it air-dry. It's a natural moisturizer.) That empty bulge (better known as post-baby belly jelly) on your abdomen will feel alien. The reality of your weight gain may hit you hard. Many women feel really depressed by this, and it's completely understandable (see box 'I look and feel crappy').

But remember your body has had an extraordinary experience; now you must focus on nurturing it and your child. You can always get back into a disciplined weight and exercise regimen at the right time once your doctor has cleared you. We can all create healthy and fit bodies for ourselves by managing our diets and exercise. Be patient. You can return to your pre-pregnancy body.

All of this might make you feel these early days are all gloom. They aren't! Most moms also remember these days as being some of the most beautiful and intense of their lives. As you watch your little one asleep in your arms, bathe them gently and nervously, laugh as they pee and poop on you, try and sing them to sleep, you'll feel emotions you never knew. Some moms say they want to shut the world out at this time and just be with their baby. It's easy to see why. Spend as much time with your baby as you can; it's your little world.

Finally, if you notice small bloodstains in your baby's diaper or slightly swollen breasts (definitely don't try to squeeze the swelling out), you may get scared and alarmed. Your baby is still coping with all the hormones you had in your body. It will settle on its own. Speak to your paediatrician about this.

(With inputs from Dr Neeru Vithalani, Dr Rita Shah and Dr Vishal Sawant)

Help! I can't breastfeed

Most moms find it difficult to breastfeed in the initial days. His neck keeps dropping off from my arm, you might wail! You may also find that your baby goes off to sleep in your arms the minute he is brought to feed. In the hospital, the nurses will give you feedback, adjust your posture, and guide your breast into the baby's mouth correctly as you feed. You might feel that you'll never get the hang of it. Or you might get into the groove easily.

Remember a few tips: like, feed your baby on demand (breast milk flow works on demand and supply, i.e., the more milk you take out, the more your body makes) and work on a proper latch (how your baby attaches to your breast) while you still have professional help and guidance at the hospital. Many moms find a feeding pillow very useful as it supports the baby so you can relax into the feeding a bit more.

After the first few days, many moms get the hang of things. On the other hand, for many moms the feeding stress increases as your baby starts to take in more milk. Typical problems are: (a) baby falling asleep at the breast and taking a long time to finish, (b) baby crying because he can't get enough milk, (c) baby getting hungry for another feed very fast, (d) finding feeding painful. Exhaustion, stress, not feeding the baby enough (you should be feeding the baby 8 to 12 feeds daily), poor feeding posture or having a premature baby are some of the main factors why women have breastfeeding troubles.

However, many women do also have low supply. According to the WHO and Unicef-published Global Breastfeeding Scorecard of 2017, worldwide only about 40 per cent of babies under six months old are exclusively breastfed.

There are many excellent breastfeeding sites to get more

advice and knowledge around these issues. However, when you have a hungry, crying infant and are battling exhaustion, it might be challenging to try and pinpoint what's going wrong.

There are now lactation consultants in most hospitals and freelance consultants in most big cities. Don't feel shy about calling an expert once you go home. A consultant will help you try different positions that will work best for you and baby, adjust your posture, help your baby latch properly and, above all, give you moral support. Feeding is not necessarily a natural process for all moms, and having a good teacher helps.

We know moms who have struggled in their first month and, after working with a consultant, gone on to feed their child for over a year! There are also many mothers who, after struggling to breastfeed their babies, eventually get down to using a breast pump to express, store and bottle-feed their breast milk for months.

Not being able to feed your child might make you feel very emotional. Many moms feel guilt and sadness. Remember there are many women who have gone through the same thing you have and that there is help available. Most importantly, if you do find feeding difficult and choose to supplement your breast milk with formula or move to formula completely, it's absolutely fine. There are excellent formulas available in the local market. Mothers beat themselves up about not doing enough for their baby (welcome to the world of parenthood!), but this is the time to be kind to yourself. If there is one message this book has, it's to give up your guilt.

Do remember that, on an average, it could take 24 to 48 hours or more post birth for your breasts to fill with milk. A lot of mothers become teary-eyed with worry because they are too anxious about using formula feeds. Neolacta is commercially available pasteurized human milk (breast milk). Talk to your paediatrician in advance about this. It is an expensive option but it is a possible option to bear in mind – even for preterm babies. It requires refrigeration, so your hospital may need to order this for you.

There are many sites to give you deeper information about breastfeeding and listings of lactation consultants in India. Here are a few:

- The Association of Lactation Professionals India (ALPI) has a listing of lactation consultants across the country and also explanations of qualifications that its listed consultants hold. Check out www.lactationprofessionalsindia.com
- Breastfeeding Support for Indian Mothers (BSIM): This is an award-winning Facebook group that has evolved into an NGO, with a presence outside of Facebook as well. Check out http://www.bsim.org.in/find-an-lc.html
- Kellymom: One of the best American websites which provides evidence-based information on breastfeeding. This was a favourite of our editor who managed to feed both her kids with the help of lactation consultants and many visits to this site. Check out https://kellymom.com
- Le Leche League (LLL): This is the best-known global NGO on breastfeeding. It has an India support page. LLL lists both lactation consultants and leaders trained to provide mother-to-mother support. Check out https://www.lllasia. org/lll-support-in-india.html

I know I am not alone in this. Many new moms go through it. Nursing your baby feels like an all-encompassing component of motherhood. You question yourself; you're crushed with self-doubt. I think, like me, most new moms don't sleep for days. My mother would tell me, 'Stay calm, eat well, relax and sleep.' You need to hear comforting words like that – from your husband, your family, your friends. Here, at this point of time, let it come from me! I have two very dear friends who have had surrogate children. Do they love their babies less because they're not putting them to the boob? I think every woman needs to balance it out. If you can breastfeed, go for it. There is no question that breast milk has so many health advantages, but don't let the pressure get to you. Sometimes the fear is debilitating. I went through this with Taimur – where I was completely dry for a good two weeks before I started lactating even a little. And I think I drove myself to distraction with the stress and pressure.

Peripartum depression

With Dr Prabha Chandra, MD, FRCPE, FRCPsych, FAMS; professor of psychiatry and in-charge of perinatal psychiatry service at NIMHANS

At the very outset, I want to clarify that while PPD is a common condition, most women can be helped and will recover. However, it is really important for women and families to know what are the normal mood variations post delivery, when to seek help and what is PPD or PPA.

The postpartum period is quite challenging for most women. The reasons are many. Lack of sleep, fatigue related to pregnancy and childbirth, meeting the demands of an infant (especially frequent breastfeeding) and the overall feeling of being responsible for a baby can be quite overwhelming. This can get compounded if women don't have enough childcare support, no support with household chores, the infant has poor health, the woman has had a difficult pregnancy, breastfeeding doesn't go as planned or there is marital conflict or interpersonal problems with other family members. Sometimes critical comments about the infant's gender or the infant's weight and looks can add to the stress. Many women are expected to follow postpartum rituals which include restrictions on food, going out or exercise. While some traditional rituals may be meaningful, many women find too many restrictions to be stressful and prevent them from finding some 'me time' in an otherwise hectic period.

Now, let's look at what we mean by perinatal mood and anxiety disorders. The most common condition is PPD. It usually happens within three months after delivery. Up to 20 per cent of mothers are seen to have PPD, and 15 per cent may have PPA. Mothers may feel sad for no reason and have crying spells. They may not feel very enthusiastic about the baby. Mums often report having negative thoughts that something bad may happen to the baby or to them. Some mothers may report a lack of feeling towards the infant, and this may be too difficult for them to express, as mothers are supposed to feel intense love towards their baby.

The signs? Family members may notice that the new mother is listless and dull, not interacting with the baby, she may not be able to concentrate and may also feel stressed and on edge. For most mothers, these feelings will be quite transient and brief and may pass on their own. However, some mothers may find that these feelings persist for more than a couple of weeks and interfere with their daily life. That's when we think that the mum needs help. So, if the new mother is unable to cheer herself up, appears dull and listless, cries easily, is irritable and feels easily overwhelmed, this may indicate PPD. Some mothers are unable to sleep, but this may often happen due to feeding schedules.

PPA occurs quite commonly alongside a low mood. Anxious

thoughts about the baby's well-being, about her own health and worries whether the breastfeeding is going well are common. However, these can become excessive, and the mind may become preoccupied with anxious thoughts that go round and round like a loop. Mothers may report that they cannot relax and always feel on edge. When does a mother need to seek help? When the low mood or anxiety persists for longer than a week continuously, when she finds it difficult to look after herself or the baby, when her appetite becomes very low, she has frequent crying spells or appears withdrawn.

PPD must be differentiated from PPA in which anxiety symptoms dominate, such as worrying a lot, inability to relax and being on edge. It must also be differentiated from postpartum blues, which is a very common problem, occurs in nearly 50–60 per cent of mums and usually happens in the first couple of weeks after childbirth. Blues are transient. Mums usually have mild mood swings which resolve within a few days. PPD must also be further differentiated from a more serious condition called postpartum psychosis, in which the mother may start hearing voices, have odd thoughts or become suspicious and irritable. If a mother has any signs of psychosis, she should immediately consult a psychiatrist as it can worsen quite rapidly and will need more detailed assessment.

So, who is at risk of PPD? Mothers who might have had depression in the past have a high chance of a recurrence during the postpartum period. It is important to discuss any previous history of mental health problems with the ob-gyn to make a care plan so that one can avoid a recurrence. Women who have poor support or have marital problems are another group that are vulnerable to depression. Also, mothers who have had a negative state of mind/mood in pregnancy have been found to worsen postpartum. Some mothers may have a negative childbirth experience because of poor obstetric care, which may also contribute to depression.

What can we do about it? Being alert to early symptoms of changes in mood is important. Encouraging a mother to talk about how she is feeling and assuring her that this will help can be very comforting. Support is very important, and the partner and family should understand that it is not her fault and that she is not being 'difficult' or 'dramatic'. Exploring how she is feeling, helping her with childcare and encouraging her to seek help are what she needs.

Is it a treatable condition? Indeed it is treatable. Milder forms of perinatal mood disorders can be helped by counselling and self-care. When the mother is not able to look after her baby, feels low or anxious most of the time and finds it difficult to function, she might need more specialist care and medication. She need not be worried about the effect of medications on the infant if she is breastfeeding as many of the antidepressants and anti-anxiety drugs are quite safe for breastfeeding.

How can partners help? Partners need to be understanding and listen, they need to help and support. Getting up at night and helping in infant care can be a big thing. It also ensures that the mother gets some sleep. Encourage the mother to take a short walk, to watch or read interesting or humorous videos or books, help her to play with the infant and allow her to express her feelings. This goes a long way towards recovery.

What is the role of a psychologist? Psychologists offer different types of therapy to women with PPD which have been found useful and have good quality evidence. These include Cognitive Behaviour Therapy and Interpersonal Therapy. They also handle issues related to any trauma in the past which might often surface during childbirth and could also contribute to bonding problems.

What is the role of a psychiatrist? A psychiatrist will assess if the PPD, blues or PPA (or any other problem like OCD or psychosis) requires medication and will prescribe the safest medication possible for the mother–infant duo. Most medications are fairly safe but need to be taken only under the supervision of a psychiatrist. And the infant should be carefully monitored for any side effects.

We should remember that talking openly about mental health is important. We must overcome the stigma related to it and not think of it as a weakness or a deficit in the mom, but consider it as something that is treatable and manageable.

Finally, here is a list of the most reliable resources to tap for peripartum depression:

- The National Institute of Mental Health and Neurosciences (NIMHANS) in Bengaluru is a premier medical institution and centre for mental health operating under the Ministry of Health and Family Welfare. NIMHANS has a 24x7 perinatal mental health helpline: +91 81057 11277. You can also email Dr Prabha Chandra at chandra@nimhans.ac.in and ask for her help in finding local resources.
- White Swan Foundation for Mental Health is a not-for-profit organization that offers knowledge-led solutions in the area of mental health by collaborating with mental health experts, persons with live experiences, like-minded individuals and organizations across the world. Its website

www.whiteswanfoundation.org has some great resources in different languages.
- Check out Postpartum Support International on www.postpartum.net and choose India to find a list of local therapists/doctors who can guide you.
- Speak to your ob-gyn to guide you to a reliable psychiatrist or psychologist.
- Speak to your local private or government hospital to connect you to their empanelled or consulting mental health practitioners.

I LOOK AND FEEL CRAPPY!

With Sonali Gupta, clinical psychologist

This thought can come to you at any time during your nine months, as you deal with your changing body and even post delivery. A pregnancy is a good realistic example of how your body is changing and what you can do about it but also of understanding what you can't do about it.

How you feel about your body rests on what has your relationship with your body been? During pregnancy, some moms feel worse, some feel fuller and more voluptuous. Maybe take a moment and ask yourself how you feel about your own self and your body at this stage.

Before your pregnancy commences, speak to your doctor. He/She will give you the best advice on what to expect in the context of how your body might change in the months to come. I have always noticed one consistent thread through my counselling sessions: that most women think they are the only one struggling with body image concerns.

However, it's very common, and many women struggle with how their body is changing.

Here is something that may help:

1. It's normal to feel jealous and to feel others have it so right. Choose to not 'blame' yourself for how your body is changing and learn to develop a healthy relationship with your body.

2. Catch yourself if you find you are engaging in a pattern of obsessive weight checking post pregnancy or even during pregnancy. It can be anxiety causing.

3. Your last trimester can be particularly hard because of how much your body changes, but enlist the support of your partner, family and friends. Honest conversations are important and go a long way and provide social soothing.

4. Relationship with social media during pregnancy: You may need to ask yourself what's the relationship you want to have with social media during your pregnancy and after. If it exhausts you and makes you anxious, figure out if you want to get off it or use it minimally and mindfully. There are many women who choose *not* to have a gaze on themselves during this time.

5. Work towards a healthy image: It's a time where you may have cravings and at the same time you may find yourself worrying over your body and putting on weight. This, in turn, can impact your mood. It's a good idea to consult your gynaecologist and speak to him/her about it. If body image concerns continue to overwhelm you and lead to excessive anxiety and low moods, speak to a mental health professional.

PART III

GETTING READY FOR THE BABY: YOUR DEFINITIVE GUIDE TO SHOPPING AND PLANNING FOR THE NURSERY

My baby preparations

Of course I went overboard during my first pregnancy! With Taimur, I bought thirty onesies, three toothbrushes, five towels and extras of everything. For one little baby! On top of that I got so many baby items as gifts.

I see now that it was such a waste. I didn't have space for most of it and I eventually ended up passing things on to my friends. With Jeh, I didn't fuss about the shopping part but focused instead on his beautiful nursery in our new house.

It is a small space – pretty tiny in fact. But it is all heart. We hand-picked everything. And it was ready well before I delivered him. Taimur's nursery in our old home was designed by my sister's best friend from Delhi. This new one for Jeh was designed by one of our friends, ex-model turned interior designer Tapur Chatterji. Both nurseries are similar. For both, I kept the colours neutral because I didn't know if I was having a boy or a girl.

Both my boys' rooms have fun wallpaper. I asked Taimur to pick the wallpaper for Jeh's room. You can imagine what he said! I guess all kids love animals. The wallpaper in Taimur's room has tigers in a South African jungle with the moon shining while his baby brother's has cheetahs and panthers on it.

Jeh's nursery is very English and a little vintage. It has hints of green and off-white with dark wood flooring and subtle pastel grey walls. There is a collage of personal family photos of Saif, Taimur and me on one wall. I got the changing table and drawers crafted in wood because it is simple, hardy and works well in any room. Baby Mozart or Baby Beethoven is always playing softly in the nursery. I think music is key to soothing babies, and adults too.

Saif wanted us to design a nursery where he would genuinely like to come every evening and just unwind with a book while the baby slept. So we have two cosy olive green velvet wing chairs and a footstool for the room. I sit there and feed Jeh and really feel at peace. The nursery truly has that energy.

I was sensible with my second pregnancy shopping. I didn't go crazy! I bought five or six onesies, four to five vests, two swaddles, two towels, one blanket and one basic oral and nail care kit. Of course I was excited to buy him some new things. But, yes, I am using most of Taimur's hand-me-downs for Jeh. There's nothing wrong with hand-me-downs! Growing up, I was given my sister's hand-me-downs all the time.

It's not just clothes. Jeh uses Taimur's old cot. It was designed by Saif and me a few months before Taimur was born. It is ivory in colour and was designed with the Pataudi crest on it. It still looks brand new. So why not reuse it, right? He is also using his big brother's baby blankets, bottle warmer and sterilizer. I never discarded any of Taimur's baby stuff. I knew I wanted a second child. And I was very sure I would use Taimur's things for my second child, whether it was a boy or a girl.

Taimur's touch-and-feel baby books – in fact every book that I have ever read to him – were all kept in cartons. They were all pulled out before Jeh was born and were dusted, cleaned, organized and set up in his nursery. I remember I used black-

and-white infant flashcards for Taimur and I am now already using some of those for Jeh. One thing I did buy afresh was a couple of sets of cot sheets and this adorable new cot mobile with baby parachutes and baby elephants on it (but that too because Taimur's cot mobile broke).

I toiled through my last two months to set up our new house well before I delivered my second baby. I felt so happy, so settled. I think being prepared really helps. I felt a lot more calm and centred when I had my home, my shopping, my nursery and my essentials in place.

6

THE ULTIMATE PREGNANCY SHOPPING LIST

Shopping can feel daunting when you are pregnant. You and your partner are constantly being given advice about what to buy by friends and baby sites, and it might feel terribly confusing, especially when you are also tired out from the pregnancy. Don't stress. What follows is the most thorough and practical list you and your partner can use – based on the experiences and feedback of many, many new moms. These are the things that really work.

If you're superstitious about shopping for your baby before her birth, give your shopping list to a trusted family member, your partner or a friend and have them shop for you as soon as you deliver your baby.

Wherever possible, optimum quantities have been recommended – assuming this is one baby. Remember if you have twins, you will need to up your quantities by double or a third – depending on your preference. So, let's break this down.

Personal items for you

This is a list of things you may use, in anticipation of your immediate needs post delivery. You can keep it ready at hand, before you go to the hospital.

- Button-down shirts/pyjama tops that you can nurse in easily and comfortable elastic waist pants for at least a month post delivery.
- *Four to five cotton nursing bras:* These are special bras with a flap that opens out and allows you to feed your baby easily. They are often softer and better padded.
- *Eight larger-sized cotton underwear:* For all those days where you will be bleeding, feeling puffy and may have itchy stitches. Some moms also pick up disposable maternity underwear. (This might be handy during your hospital stay though.)
- *Two packets of cotton (non-synthetic) sanitary napkins to start with:* Non-synthetic surfaces really help in the beginning when you may be dealing with stitches. Later, you can switch to your regular sanitary napkins.
- *One nipple soothing ointment:* If you prefer a home remedy, a lot of women keep washed and dried cabbage leaves in the refrigerator to tuck into their bra to soothe sore nipples while nursing.
- *One set of disposable breast pads:* To insert in your bra for leaky breasts. Don't buy too many to start with. There is a chance you may not need these at all.
- *A breastfeeding pillow:* This is not necessary, but a lot of moms find this indispensable. It might help to keep an additional slip cover.
- *A nursing blanket or apron:* This is optional, in case you need to cover yourself if you're feeding in front of someone.
- Your preferred oil for postnatal massages.
- *Abdominal support belt:* This is optional and it helps to support your weakened back and your loose abdominal muscles. Many families traditionally use a nine-yard saree to wrap around your abdomen for a few hours every morning. In the case of a

vaginal birth, you can use a saree, corset or belt as soon as you're home from the hospital. Moms with C stitches have to wait.

Feeding the baby

Most moms say that apart from the fear of labour, their next biggest fear is breastfeeding. It's very common for moms – first-time moms especially – to feel stressed about this and guilty if they are not managing to get their feeding right. Science will tell you that breast milk is best for the baby, but it's not always possible for moms to manage. Whatever happens, do not feel guilty and beat yourself up about it. This is not the time for it, and moreover your baby has plenty of excellent options for nutrition. Do what you can! You might breastfeed your baby exclusively or choose to supplement her with formula feeds. Some moms choose to pump their breast milk and bottle-feed it to their baby. Others just move purely to formula feed.

- *Three to eight bottles:* There are many excellent baby bottles available in the market. Pick ones made of BPA-free plastic. Most of the bottles are sold for particular ages (0–3 months, 3–6 months, etc.) and will come with age-appropriate nipples. So be aware of this and check the bottle description carefully to see what age the nipple is for. Does it really make a difference to give a newborn a nipple for a six-month-old? Not really. The nipples vary by how fast and slow the milk flows through them – slow-flow nipples are recommended for the newborn so they don't get used to a fast flowing bottle and then refuse the breast. An older baby who is used to feeding can take a faster flowing nipple.

  Bottles come in approximate 4 oz and 8 oz sizes. The 8 oz ones will last you till the baby is at least one-plus, but a smaller bottle might be useful in the early stages. Remember, your baby will need feeding between six to eight times for the first few months, and it's useful to get enough bottles so you are not always washing them. For moms who will just supplement breast milk with bottle feeds, three bottles of 8 oz might be enough. For those who are doing exclusive bottle feeding, consider at least six. Many moms go for eight bottles, but you can find your optimum number as you go along.

- *A baby bottle sterilizer:* If your baby is using a bottle, then these need to be sterilized for every feed. You can do this on the stove-top, but cheap and effective sterilizers are available today. These are either microwave or electric and sold in different sizes. If your baby will be primarily bottle-fed, you should pick a bigger one.

  Note: There are now plastic sterilizer bags available to take with you on a trip.

- *Bottle cleaning station:* It's useful having a small corner set aside in the kitchen/baby room as your bottle station. You might want to have a closed plastic box to store cleaned and sterilized bottles in this station, plus an open plastic bowl where dirty bottles are stored. This is where the sterilizer can be kept too.

- *Bottle cleaning apparatus:* You will need one baby bottle cleaning brush, one nipple cleaning brush and one baby bottle washing liquid. The brushes might even come with the bottle.

- *A bottle warmer (i.e., a small machine that gently warms your baby's milk bottle):* This may be pretty handy if you are bottle-feeding – it can be used to warm breast milk and formula feeds. If you don't want one, you can also warm the milk bottle in a wide mug filled with freshly boiled water.

- *Electric kettle:* You may already have this at home. You'll find it comes handy for all kinds of tasks as mentioned above.
- *A traditional Indian long-nozzled steel 'chamach' (i.e., bondula):* To feed your baby any SOS medicines or even for early top feeds of formula (this is because many people don't want to put the baby on a bottle early on).
- Three soft cloth bibs – especially if you plan to use a bottle or the 'chamach'.
- *One box of newborn/infant formula:* Many moms will choose to formula-feed or find they need to supplement breast milk, so it's worth keeping a box with you in any case. Ask your paediatrician and friends/family who have delivered recently to figure out which brand to go with. (P.S.: You may also go through a short trial-and-error phase to figure out which formula is suitable for your baby.) Store your formula in an airtight box.
  Note: Speak to your paediatrician about Neolacta, commercially available pasteurized human milk (see section 'Help! I can't breastfeed' in Chapter 5: Your First Two Weeks after Delivery).
- *One breast pump and two hands-free pumping bras:* Again, this is optional. Here your breasts are pumped with the help of a machine and breast milk is collected in an attached feeding bottle. It's useful for moms who are returning to work and want their babies to get breast milk while they are out of the house, for moms who want to bottle-feed the baby but with breast milk, or even if you have a preemie who is stuck in the NICU for weeks, away from you. It is also very useful if you want to stimulate the process of lactation early on in the hospital or if your breasts are engorged.

  Breast pumps come in manual and electric options. If you know that you will be pumping regularly, all moms will tell you that you will need to go electric. A machine will remove milk from you much faster and more effectively. Do note, however, that these are expensive. The hand pump is significantly cheaper, but using it can be a slow and tiring process.

If you do plan to make pumping a regular part of your life, then you must invest in a hands-free pumping bra, which will let you pump without having to hold the bottles. This will help make the whole process much more relaxing. Buy two as you'll find that the bra will need to be washed pretty frequently.

- If you plan to pump (i.e., express) and freeze your milk, you will need a set of breast milk storage freezer bags.

Baby care

- *30–40 newborn-size diapers and/or 12 reusable cloth nappies:* Diapers are indispensable but they are very damaging to the environment, causing a great deal of landfill. Remember to buy the newborn size.

  There is now a move among many moms to return to the old-fashioned cloth nappies. Do note these definitely need more care, and it might feel like something outside your current bandwidth. Above all, you need to be relaxed and stress-free through this journey, so pick what suits you. If you are going cloth, then pick nappies with Velcro sides or press buttons (don't opt for strings or safety pin options). Many moms choose to use cloth nappies in the day and diapers overnight.

  Tip: Moms have found 'nappy pads' an invaluable accompaniment to cloth nappies.

- *Six to eight soft napkins:* For multipurpose uses – as you'll be constantly wiping your baby clean, dabbing her clothes or even sponging her with these.
- *12 muslin napkins, roughly about 30 cm x 30 cm (i.e., 100 per cent cotton muslin napkins):* These are incredibly versatile. It's a soft, absorbent and breathable large-sized napkin (comes in plain colours, white or prints) that works as a temporary bib, washcloth and/or burp cloth. If you have a particularly dexterous nurse, jhappa maid or grandmom, she may be able to fashion this napkin into a temporary nappy too!
- *A basic care kit with nail clippers and hairbrush is enough:* A baby toothbrush is only used later; you will be cleaning your newborn baby's gums with soft gauze or soft cloth dipped in boiled and cooled water.
- *One each of a baby body wash (liquid), baby shampoo and baby lotion:* Look for products that are sulphate- and paraben-free. There are home-grown Indian organic baby products available in the market today, and almost all the popular international baby brands are easily available too. Finding products that work for your baby may also be a short trial-and-error process. Do bear in mind that paediatricians actively discourage the use of baby dusting powders and eye kajal.
  Note: For the first few days, till the umbilical cord falls off, you won't be using any soap on your baby's body.
- *One or two receiving blankets (to carry the baby):* Thick or thin depending on the time of year. This is really just a simple, squarish blanket (sometimes hooded). Moms use it to take their babies out of the house. A simple thin dohar would also work here. This is an optional buy.
- *Three to four swaddle cloths:* This is a large piece of soft fabric you can use to swaddle the baby, or it can double up as a

light blanket. Many moms prefer cotton chaddars, or dohars. Some like fitted jersey swaddles. It's your call. But you will need a slightly large soft cloth for swaddling in the first few months.

- *Alcohol-free wet wipes, sterilized cotton and cotton buds:* Wet wipes will be your best friend for a long, long time, even after your little baby has grown up and can walk and talk. You could also use them to clean your baby's potty, though you may just use water with sterilized cotton. Ask your paediatrician to guide you towards cleaning your baby's genitals.
- *A foldable 'travel' changing mat:* Many moms buy an additional foldable changing mat for when they are out with the baby.
- *A diaper bag:* Try as hard as you can to avoid it, but you will need a dedicated baby bag. Why are these so handy? The slots, of course! These magic bags have pockets for wet wipes, diapers, extra clothes, changing mats, feeding bottles and much more.
- *Baskets or a simple big tray for your baby's toiletries:* This will help keep all of these things organized.

Baby clothes and laundry

- *Three to five thin inner vests – i.e., ganjis/bundis:* If you live in cooler climates or if it's winter, consider thicker vests.
- *Three to five rompers, which are full-length and full-sleeved bodysuits:* These are especially useful for the night (adjust the quantity if you plan to use pyjama sets for the night).
- *Three to five half onesies, which are half-sleeved and end at the diaper:* These are great for warm weather and when you want your baby to get some sun or just play.
- *Four sets of comfortable pyjama sets for the baby to sleep in:* Especially in case you don't want to use the bodysuits.

- *Four to five tops which are either front snap or side snap or kimono style*: It is tougher to slip on T-shirts from the baby's head. For summer babies, good old Indian jhablas are just great. These are thin, soft and super easy to use. Keep four of these jhablas, at the very least. These are specifically handy during the time your baby's umbilical cord hasn't fallen off.
- *Three to five elasticized waist pants and/or shorts:* You can slip these on under the half onesies too.
- *Three to four pairs of socks or booties and two pairs of mittens:* Mittens are so that your baby doesn't scratch her face when not swaddled. Baby nails can be sharp and long at birth and tend to grow quickly.

  Note: If you plan to dress your baby in full-length onesies for most of the time (some of which come with attached mittens), you won't need these two items.
- *Two caps:* Opt for cotton ones.
- *A mild infant washing detergent (hypoallergenic if you're fussy) and an antiseptic fluid like Dettol or Savlon (optional; and only if you prefer):* This is for the baby's clothes, napkins, sheets, etc. Having said that, bear in mind that a simple liquid detergent meant for adult clothes will also do for your baby's clothes. Many moms opt to keep a fabric softener – but this is entirely optional. If your baby's clothes are going in the washing machine, you will be using your general washing machine detergent anyway.
- One designated baby laundry basket might be helpful – although it is optional.

  Tip: Keep a designated plastic bucket for your baby's soiled cloth nappies and so on. The soiled nappy can be rinsed off thoroughly and then left in a plastic bucket till the next day's wash.

These are the basics. Additions to this list depend on your personal preferences – like if you want a few dresses for your baby girl or dungarees for your baby boy! If you're confused about sizing, most average weight newborn babies will fit into the 0–3 month or 'NB' (i.e., newborn) size. If you have a bigger baby, she may outgrow this starter size a lot faster. You can also go conservative in your quantities in the beginning and pick up more clothes as and when you need them. In case you're wondering how warm you need to keep your baby, most paediatricians will tell you to use just one additional layer for your baby than you use for yourself.

Baby medical

- *One diaper/nappy rash ointment:* There are some moms who like to use a lighter ointment during the day and a thicker one for overnight use.
- *One nasal aspirator (rubber or tube):* Pick the manual aspirators over the electric ones. Many moms love the tube aspirators, which you have to blow out from one end. They find it is more effective in removing nasal mucus.
- One or two medicine droppers. Many moms find a baby medicine syringe most easy to handle.
- One thermometer. Forehead or ear thermometers which are pricier but much more useful are great options for you to consider.
- One big pump-top bottle of liquid hand sterilizer – for everyone to use before handling the baby.
- Eau de cologne or doctor-recommended spirit to keep the umbilical cord stump clean until it falls off on its own. Ask the hospital nurse to show you how to keep the umbilical cord clean.

- *Saline nasal spray:* This is very useful to clear up stuffy noses.
- *Liquid paracetamol:* You could keep infant Crocin around but, in any case, don't medicate your baby without consulting your paediatrician. In case of any other problems, let your paediatrician guide you to the right medicine.
- *Hing roll/colic medicine:* Hing roll is the traditional cure for colic, and many moms find it extremely useful to apply hing on their baby's tummy. There are also Western colic medicines such as gripe water. However, their effectiveness isn't medically proven, although they aren't considered harmful.

Baby massage and bath time

- *One bottle of oil:* Oils are traditionally picked based on the season or, at times, even cultural practices. For instance, coconut oil for a summer baby or almond oil for a winter baby. A lot of Indian and international brands have special baby massage oils too. Many Indian families also keep a small bottle of castor oil handy – this is used exclusively to press into the gentle and still semi-soft scalp (i.e., the 'soft spot') of the baby's head. If your paediatrician does not recommend massages very early on or the use of oil, wait for a bit till you rush on this. Do not commence any type of massages on your baby till your first visit to the paediatrician – which will be 8 to 10 days post birth. Your baby needs to have a healthy cord, she needs to be free of any jaundice and she should have regained the 200 grams or so that she will have lost at the time of discharge from the hospital (this is normal).
- *A baby bath tub and a bathing mug:* There are also baby bath chairs/bathers that many moms find very useful as it helps to

stabilize and support the baby while you focus on the bathing. You can also find special mugs to wash your baby's hair. Ask your paediatrician on baby bath protocol until the time her umbilical cord falls off. Most often, it is ideal to simply sponge your baby until her umbilical cord falls off on its own.

- A plastic bathroom stool is useful for the adult who is bathing the baby.
- Two soft towels with hoods.
- Two washcloths (entirely optional) – to sponge your baby.

Baby bed (if you are investing in a cot)

A good quality adjustable baby cot that can be used from day one till your child is about three years old is a single and solid investment. Here is what you'd need:

- *Two to three fitted sheets:* These are very convenient and easy to use. You should have at least two sets of cot sheets – your baby can throw up, have a diaper leak or pee at any time.
- *One to three flat sheets:* You may use these for the cot instead of fitted ones. If you are buying fitted sheets for the crib, you can skip this or buy just one.
- *One or two plastic liner/PVC sheets:* Line the mattress with a plastic liner and place the bed sheet on top. These liners come in various sizes.

  Here's a tip: Many stores have a small (think baby-sized) super handy plastic liner with two to three extra cloth liners that you can attach to the plastic with the help of four corner press buttons. This way, your baby's skin isn't touching plastic, and you don't need another extra layer of a soft sheet or napkin between the baby and the plastic sheet. When the cloth liner soils, you throw it in the wash and attach another cloth liner. This is useful for those times when you've taken off your baby's diaper for a short period of time.

- *Two thin blankets like dohars plus one thick duvet and/or blanket sacks:* Kids often kick away their blankets, and many moms find it easier to put them in a blanket sack that zips up like a sleeping bag and keeps them warm. Many moms also opt for cellular cot blankets (woven blankets with lots of very tiny closely spaced holes), to prevent any risk of suffocation.

- *Umbrella mosquito nets:* This is optional but pretty handy. It will cover the length of your baby while she sleeps.

- We love doing up cots! But do you need to? The answer is no. A baby does not need a pillow (see box 'Do you need pillows?'). A four-sided bumper for a cot is a mere cosmetic add-on. Nor does your baby need any toys in her cot. A cot bumper and toys are also dust hazards. Keep your cot minimal (see box 'SIDS'). A simple cot mobile suspended above the baby's cot is the only entertainment/toy that most moms consider.

- As you prep for the baby bed, remember to prep your own. Line your own mattress with a full-sized plastic/PVC liner and then lay your bed sheet on top. Keep a couple of extra bed sheets handy at all times. There is nothing more annoying than scrambling for a fresh sheet in the middle of the night when your baby has thrown up or her pee has leaked on your bed and you're incredibly groggy. This can happen as you feed your baby or change her diaper.

Do you need pillows?

Most paediatricians in India and across the world recommend against using any pillow for babies – at the least till the age of one or sometimes even after. Grandmoms may tell you your baby needs a pillow to be comfortable or that your newborn's misshapen head needs a pillow to correct itself. There is no scientific evidence to back this up! A simple sloped/wedge baby reflux pillow might be the only value-add here, if your baby is prone to regurgitating. Speak to your paediatrician about this pillow before you pick it up.

Optional

This is a list of items which you may not really need until the baby has crossed one to three months or more. It depends on how you plan to move with your baby, how much you plan to leave your house with your baby and how you'd like to carry your baby around.

- *Car seat:* In some countries it is legally mandated and you cannot leave the hospital without a car seat for your baby. This is not the case in India. Most new moms prefer to swaddle and carry their newborn babies in their arms during a car ride. Car seats are expensive and they also take up space in a car but they do keep your child safer. It's really worth the investment. There are special newborn car seats, but you can also get car seats that a child can use from 0 upwards till they are about eight years old (or till they weigh 18–24 kg).

Globally, parents then switch to booster seats till their kids are nearly 12 years old or weigh 40 kg.

Note: Car seats can be tricky to install, so you may have to do some practice runs to install it perfectly.

- *A carry cot or Moses basket and/or a sling baby carrier:* For the first few months, you might want to use a carry cot or Moses basket to carry the baby around. The Moses basket will allow the baby to sleep comfortably anywhere but it has a very short shelf life. A sling baby carrier (kangaroo pack or kangaroo carrier) is attached to your body as you go out and these can be used even till the child is two or three years old, depending on her weight. It is an easy, hygienic and fuss-free way to carry your child around.

- Some moms find an envelope/sleeping bag extremely convenient to use in a stroller, in your hand or even on a bed at home.

- *Pram/Stroller:* Most moms pick up a pram pre-delivery or soon after. However, it is not critical. You can also wait for one to four months or till you start taking your baby out for a stroll or travel with her to pick one up.

- *A bouncer:* A bouncer can be of great assistance when you have things to do and your little one can be securely tied to a bouncer or infant swing and gently bounced/rocked to sleep.

- *Play mat/Play gym:* A play gym is essentially a soft mat with two arches on which a bunch of toys dangle – with lights, textures, mirrors and kick-activated music. It is very cute, but your baby won't exactly care much for it in the very beginning. You could easily choose to wait for a bit (one to two months) before you invest in one. This is a good buy once your baby is observing things, trying to grab things and can lift her neck and see what's around during tummy playtime.

- *A bed railing:* If you plan to put your baby down on a regular bed for naps and playtime, do not skip the side railing. After the first five months of her life, your baby will wriggle and turn over. Babies falling off the side of beds are one of the most common baby accidents.

7

PLANNING FOR THE NURSERY

Somewhere through your pregnancy you and your partner will start considering your baby's nursery. Now, is it always a designated baby room? Of course not. Not everyone has a spare bedroom or den in their home that can be converted into a dedicated baby nursery! You and your partner can also carve out a corner of your own bedroom for your baby and make it work. As we go over each aspect of a nursery, you will find options for both.

Where should the nursery be?

If you're doing up a new nursery, pick a room with a window. And if you're going to be improvising a baby corner in your bedroom, do make sure it is not against a window. Why? Harsh sunlight and – just – because you're a mom – you'll constantly think about the hazards of a window.

The basics of a nursery

Now, if you're doing up a nursery – the world is your canvas. You can get the flooring of your choice (many moms prefer wood), paint the ceiling bright and use wallpaper. A wall mural can be bright and fun; there are dedicated mural artists whom you can hire. Figure out a few personal touches – like height charts, your baby's name on the wall, monogrammed bedding and so on. And definitely incorporate a bookshelf with shelves to hold large-sized picture books – you will need it for years. (My editor has a special tip: remember the shelf heights should be tall enough to accommodate large picture books. Most children's books are about A4 size.) Go for a fun gender-neutral colour. Those lacy pinks and boisterous blues may get tiresome – also, gender stereotyping, anyone? – while shades of yellow, green, powder blue or good old white are likelier to get you through the years.

Here, however, are some basics that will make your baby space user friendly:

- *Blackout curtains:* For the baby to learn to sleep through the night, one of the key things is to be able to distinguish between day and night. Blackout curtains help to keep the room very dark through the night and early morning. For moms who are planning to share the room with their baby, you can also just add a blackout lining to your curtains.

- *Dimmable lights:* Babies will require frequent night feeding and nappy changing. A dim light will be less harsh for both of you. A table light with shades is also a good option. It is best not to turn on too many lights and overstimulate your baby during night feeds and diaper changes. Having a light on your baby through the night is invaluable. One plug-in night light for the room where your baby will be sleeping is a must – whether it is a nursery or your bedroom.

- If you are designing a nursery from scratch, think about a floor that is easy to clean, durable and reasonably low maintenance. Carpets and rugs look super cute, but are quite a dust hazard.

Wait till your baby is older to add a carpet or rug to his space.

- *A comfortable chair:* It's very important to have a cushioned, supportive chair for when you feed your baby. Many moms love a nice armchair or rocking chair.

- When planning a nursery, account for a handy table against a wall with an accessible plug point. If your baby is going to be in your bedroom, just place a small table near a plug point. Why? You may need to plug in a sterilizer or bottle warmer, a kettle or a facial steamer in case of a nasal congestion. You never know!

- Plan the wardrobes to accommodate the growing needs of your baby. You will not refurbish this space in a hurry. If you plan your shutter space and shelving cleverly (and optimally), you won't have a clutter of clothes, toiletries or toys for a good few years. If you're getting a special wardrobe for the baby and customizing it for him, don't forget the rods. Your baby has tiny clothes but he will soon have things to hang neatly on hangers. A good tip is to try – as far as possible – to have all storage in shutters (i.e., enclosed).

- Buy one medium-sized, lidded and wide-mouthed dustbin to throw soiled diapers in. You want a lid to trap the smells, and a wide mouth means you can easily chuck the diapers in. Those cute small chrome bins used in bathrooms fill up super fast. Line a lidded bin with a regular dustbin liner and you're good to go. Some moms opt for a dedicated diaper genie (i.e., a special diaper bin that has a tight lid). You can also use biodegradable nappy sacks (these often come in packs of 50 or 100 – so keep one to start with) to place the potty-soiled diapers in.

- *Baby monitor:* These come in audio-only and audio/video options. It is optional. But if you are pottering around the house, and your baby is asleep in a separate room, you will feel more at ease if you have an ear out for him. This is a single and solid purchase that is a proper value-add. You can catch many accidents and untoward incidents with regard to your baby via this one audio-visual baby monitor.

- And the big and invaluable one! A changing table (or changing station). A changing station is the dedicated spot where you change the baby's diapers and clothes – usually a firm surface with at least 32 inches (or roughly 2.5 feet) of usable space on top and at the approximate height of an average dining table. It's also where you keep all the stuff your baby will need: diapers, nappy creams, napkins, swaddles and everyday clothes. Remember – everything you need to change your baby should be at grabbing distance. You are not going to want to leave your baby unattended on a table for even a second as you go hunting for something.

  Ideally, the changing table top has an edging; some ready ones come with short safety railings. Do ensure you pick something sturdy – whether ready, custom-made or refurbished, there should be no tipping threat. Changing tables can have a set of drawers or simple open shelving below. If you have the space/budget, go all out and get a fully equipped changing table with drawers and storage space. Many moms have repurposed furniture into changing tables, from office desks to a chest of drawers at the right height. You can, of course, use your bed to change the baby, but you'll discover that changing a baby can be a messy affair!

- A changing table will need a changing mat on top. The foam changing mats that are a bit spongy and soft work really well. Ask at the store if the changing pad you're buying has additional changing pad covers – if yes, about three of these might be helpful. This changing mat can be moved to the bed or floor too, as required, to change your baby. Many companies make changing mats with a safety strap.

The baby bed

Your baby might be sleeping in a cot next you or in his own room. Whether it is a nursery or your own bedroom, let your baby's bed be away from a window. It is ideal that your baby does not share your bed with you at any point of time.

Cot/Crib: A crib is a baby bed with rails, which can be used typically till the child is three or even four. This is a single, solid and highly recommended investment for any mom. You do also get mini cribs, though that is a rather short-term option.

- Pick a cot where one side can go up and down, allowing you to pick up your baby easily. However be vigilant – lowered rails are a definite hazard, so you want them up as soon as possible.
- Many moms find it useful to either buy a cot with lockable wheels or get a set of four lockable wheels added by a local carpenter. This way, you have the flexibility of moving your baby to another room if needed.
- Some moms find it useful to pick up a cot with a net covering or get a customized net covering made.
- The American Academy of Pediatrics (AAP) says that a baby should be put to sleep without anything loose in the bed – no pillows of any kind, soft toys, loose blankets or crib liner. In India, the culture is different. You will most likely be gifted at least one bedding set, which will typically come with two side pillows and a head pillow. Should you use it? Current

medical advice says no, although this will upset the more traditional members of your family! Always speak to your paediatrician if you have any doubts about pillows (see box 'Do you need pillows?').

Co-sleeping

Every doctor will advise you to keep your baby in the same room if you need to, but not on the same bed as you. If space is tight, what are your choices then?

Bassinet

A bassinet – which is a bed for up to four-month-old babies – is smaller than a cot. If you have bought a Moses basket as a baby carrying device, it can double up as your baby cot for a short time. The con is that it will mean yet another purchase once the baby has outgrown it. Also note that the typical crib/cot sheets on sale may be too large for a bassinet.

Co-sleeping crib

Look up co-sleeping cribs or cots. It's a great option for your baby to sleep next to your bed, in his own space. These cribs have a railing on only three sides (rather than four) and can basically be lined up right against your bed. However, paediatricians will advise you to put your baby to sleep at least five to six feet away from you. It ensures better sleep for you, it is safer for your baby and it reduces your baby's co-dependency on you from an early stage. Also the same point holds here as for the bassinet – you will need to eventually move to a proper size crib, so it means a second purchase.

SIDS

SIDS or sudden infant death syndrome is a very frightening but extremely rare occurrence. Also known as 'cot death', it is the sudden and unexplained death of an infant (one year or younger, usually between one and six months) and it generally happens in the baby's sleep. There are no specific reasons that can make a baby susceptible to SIDS – though research shows male babies are more at risk than females. SIDS most often remains unexplained, despite medical analyses and autopsies. But the feeling of guilt and trauma to the family is overwhelming.

There are a few factors that seem to be indicative of the risk of SIDS, starting with the likeliest cause: (1) a hidden issue like a brain development abnormality or maturational delay (a problem in neuro-regulation or cardio-respiratory control); (2) low birth weight or preterm babies; (3) a very soft bed; (4) sleeping on the side or on the stomach; (5) exposure to second-hand smoke; (6) overheating the baby (i.e., keeping the baby way warmer than needed); (7) hereditary (if there is a family history of SIDS).

Some of the important precautions for SIDS (which are also great for the overall well-being and care of your baby) are: (1) putting the baby to sleep on his back; (2) using a good mattress (i.e., a firm one); (3) keeping the baby cot/bed free of pillows, toys, padding and thick quilts; (4) keeping a close watch on the baby till at least six months of age; (5) sharing a room with your baby if you need to, but not sharing the same bed; (6) keeping your baby propped up or making sure he burps before you put him down to sleep after a full feed (more so if it's a formula feed).

(With inputs from Dr Neeru Vithalani)

PART IV

NUTRITION, FITNESS AND SELF-CARE

8

NUTRITION
With Rujuta Diwekar

My pregnancy eating

You'll know by now that my two pregnancies were completely different from each other. But there was one common strand that ran through both of them – my obsession with pepperoni pizza! I am not into pepperoni at all usually. When not pregnant, I love being vegetarian. But I got ravenous for meat while pregnant and craved cold cuts, salt and soy. It was as if I was another person.

Whenever we went out with friends, it was a given that I would eat pepperoni pizza. During Taimur's time, the feasting was at my favourite local restaurant, Out of the Blue. My friends would sit across the table from me – watching in disbelief (and probably embarrassment) as I demolished one pizza after another. I was a content, belching, pizza-guzzling star. When I was pregnant with Jeh, we were locked down, which means it was a crazy amount of pepperoni pizza takeaway from Ray's – a pizza parlour that's five minutes from my house. Twice or thrice a week!

All that salt intake took its toll. In my last trimester during both pregnancies, I got bloaty under the eyes. My fingers swelled up so much that I couldn't take off my ring. I wisened up the second time around though and took off my rings by my eighth month. Forced to choose between my pepperoni and my wedding ring, I chose pepperoni!

Mind you, I am very health conscious usually. I never add extra salt to my homemade salad. I know it's not great for me. And if I gave into my cravings on one day, I would try to be super healthy for the next two days. But then I'd fall off the wagon again. I guess there is no pregnancy without cravings.

Now I wasn't all pizza through the nine months and did also try and eat as well as possible. When I first began working with my nutritionist Rujuta Diwekar, she got me to start the morning with a banana and I've stuck to that. It is excellent for your iron and potassium requirements. So my day always, always begins with one banana and five almonds. This has never changed, whether or not I'm pregnant.

Breakfast was typically poha, upma or two idlis. It is the most basic Indian diet – and I can't live without it. I stopped all caffeine during Taimur's time. My first pregnancy and all, right? I wanted to be '100 per cent good'. I went mostly caffeine-free again for my second pregnancy, but did have half a cup of tea in the morning. I couldn't do my morning chai during my first trimester with Jeh, though, as the sight of milk made me sick.

I made a diligent effort to stick to smaller meals (or portions), especially in my first five months during both pregnancies. During Taimur's time I must admit I mostly indulged the whole nine months. In Jeh's time I didn't feel like eating much – and this was especially pronounced during my first trimester, when

I was very nauseous. Even a glass of water would make me hurl. My appetite picked up from the sixth month on.

Food was how I bonded with my closest friends through both my pregnancies. While Taimur's time was all about eating out and travelling, my second pregnancy was a little more home-bound, owing to the pandemic. When I wasn't working, we would plan many long and elaborate lunches at one home after another where I would decide what I wanted to eat and my friends would do a potluck. One would bring her awesome sambhar, and the other would do her amazing potatoes. A chaat meal at my house would mean absolutely every favourite chaat item, made by my cook at home from scratch; nothing was store-bought!

You might think that I eat exotic, fancy food the whole time. Sushi one day, biryani on another! Well, let me tell you I am a desi girl, that too a proper Punjabi at heart. I love my Indian food and need my roti, dahi, dal, sabzi every day. That's been my lunch for years. And I am not fussy when it comes to vegetables. I eat everything from lauki and turai to karela and baingan. I especially like all my healthy greens. I always eat my greens at lunch. The only veggie I don't like eating is bhindi! It's just the boys (Saif and Tim – and Jeh eventually, I suppose) in my family who eat bhindi.

I had a lot of south Indian food cravings (like sambhar–rice or dahi–rice with grated cucumber) and did a lot of south Indian meals with friends. I also ate a lot of simple Maharashtrian dishes, such as varan-bhaat. I prefer my food cooked in mustard oil or half a tsp of homemade ghee. And I make an effort to try different oils round the year. I am very particular about my oils and ghee. Most of the food I eat is made at home by my cook. I have an excellent Nepali cook who has lived in India for most of his life.

Throughout my pregnancies, a glass of chaach or a fruit for the 4 to 6 p.m. snack craving was my thing. When I am not pregnant, fruit is never usually my snack. In fact, my mid-evening snack is a cup of coffee with banana chips and makhana. But while pregnant, I forced myself to eat that seasonal fruit. It's healthy, sure; but I also found that when I ate a fruit, I didn't miss my afternoon caffeine kick. It's a trick I used on myself, I guess!

And my tea is the proper Indian kadak chai, by the way, with half a teaspoon of sugar. My coffee is also the traditional one, with a dash of milk and sugar. I don't believe in using sugar-free alternatives. So I ended up cutting out a lot of sugar by skipping these beverage cravings. Coffee during pregnancy hasn't worked for me anyway – I literally felt my heart race and my BP shoot up.

Fortunately for me, I had no sugar cravings – except for maybe that occasional scoop of chocolate ice cream. Dessert has never been my thing. My sister, on the other hand, can sit in front of the TV with a big piece of chocolate cake and truly savour every bite. But I don't give in to sugar cravings. Nor do Saif and Taimur, for that matter. I guess we are lucky in that. My only after-dinner sweet treat – and that too not every day – would be simple homemade yogurt in which I mixed chopped dates, cashews, pistachios and raisins. It was good for me and for my baby and was great for dealing with a spot of indigestion too.

I didn't do roti–sabzi for dinner through both pregnancies. It was usually fish or chicken (with a little smattering of red meat) with rice, maybe with a vegetable side dish. I moved between brown rice, quinoa, white rice and, on occasion, pasta for dinner. It was all simple and (mostly!) healthy, except when I gave in to my pizza cravings. Nothing fancy. Just clean flavours. Olive oil, lemon and sometimes garlic were the only seasonings in my fish or meat. I was pretty good about wrapping up dinner two to three hours before going to bed. But this was in my second pregnancy, when I actually could not keep my eyes open beyond 11 p.m. The first time I was out for dinners, partying all night till 3 a.m., and entertaining extensively at home!

Saif is a really good cook. He cooked me Chinese, Thai and Malaysian and was in the kitchen twice or thrice a week, when he was not working. He did a lot of cooking during the second pregnancy in particular. The pandemic made him an even better chef! I like eating his meals because he has a light hand when it comes to seasoning and I especially love his healthy mustard chicken and a chilli chicken he makes with brown rice. This cooking habit lasts round the year, you should know – it wasn't just a special treat for his pregnant wife!

Apart from trying to eat healthy every day, I didn't have any special pregnancy food hacks. I did have one great pregnancy food – a mutton and paya soup made by my cook at home. It was a must for me during both my pregnancies, and I had it once a week, if not more. It's basically a hearty stock complete with the trotters and meat and it really strengthens the bones. As you know, a baby is predisposed to suck calcium off your bones, when it is in short supply. I was always wary about keeping my energy levels up, especially as I worked throughout both my pregnancies. I still breezed through my pregnancy with Taimur. But during Jeh's time, while the first six months were fine, from the seventh month on, I would feel myself dip post 5 p.m.

As for avoiding foods, as you know, I cut down on the caffeine. Along with this, I kept raw foods to a minimum, even though I love salads. During my pregnancies and even in the post-delivery period, I would opt for lightly cooked salads, like boiled beetroot, corn and chana. Those raw leaves really scared me! Raw foods and juices have never suited my body. In the Ayurveda tradition, my body dosha is kapha. I need to have a lot of dahi and other soothing foods. We have to understand that what suits a western body doesn't necessarily suit ours. I just went with properly cooked food made in ghee and when I felt like eating really simply, I'd go for a toast with homemade white butter or a simple bowl of ghee-rice. These are things my dadi would always recommend and they really worked for me.

Nor did I drive myself nuts and start eating and drinking foods to promote lactation (although my yogurt and khajoor recipe is good for lactation, incidentally). My mother and grandmother did try to push the third trimester and post-delivery ghee, besan and gond laddoos on me. Culturally, we have so many post-baby traditions when it comes to food. It's all really wonderful, and I know it comes from the heart and everyone means well. But the gond laddoos were too heavy for me – I just couldn't do too many laddoos or for too long!

After having Jeh and while I actively nursed him, I was very focused on eating right – I added ghee to my diet with a lot of millets. And I completely avoided spicy food. I have to admit that I did not eat exactly what I really wanted to eat or felt like eating, but I simply did what was good for my baby.

I believe it is too tough to follow a pattern set by someone else and it's best to create your own good habits that feel like something you can follow. In any case, each pregnancy will be its own journey – I say this from experience. So whenever anyone tried to lecture me – 'this is how you should eat/drink/behave' – I would just listen with one ear and take it out from the other.

While I always had Rujuta to guide me towards eating right, I did pack in a lot of calories during my pregnancy. And I know I overdid it during Taimur's time. I was 25 kg up when I delivered him. While Rujuta was firing me left, right and centre, I was busy killing it with samosas from Punjab Sweet House and many rounds of pani-puri. I was much better during Jeh's time though. I did salmon, broccoli, ghee-rice, a glass of milk at bedtime (but the pepperoni pizzas did not stop) – the kind of stuff that would make a nutritionist proud! As I've mentioned before, I am not small built; I never have been. And I never could figure out how some pregnant women only put on that belly weight. I really have to work at my body. I put on about 19 kg with Jeh. Did my doctor yell at me? Of course he did!

Bebo has been my closest friend, my soul sister, for over twenty years. We had so much fun in Taimur's time! All our outings were to a restaurant. I think I doubled in size with her and was proxy preggers. We really killed the pizzas! I vowed I would drag her to the gym post pregnancy and I did. I never gave her a day off. Through her pregnancy, she had it all – pasta, pizza, an occasional glass of wine – everything she had been disciplined about earlier. No one's opinions mattered to her. We had extended lunches that went on to dinner. While she would eat lunch, she was already deciding her dinner – and her next day's breakfast and lunch too! That is how much she enjoyed letting go. She didn't give a toss about her appearance, nor did she think twice about what people expect of her. She would burp constantly and had swollen feet from all the high-salt food she was eating. But that never stopped her from running for food! She loved my mom's fish curry and would come home just for that. She'd show up at another friend's house to eat Gujarati thali. Her second pregnancy was different and a lot quieter. We spent many long hours over potluck meals at home. Despite her weight gain, her face always stayed lean – so with a slightly cheating

camera angle and loose clothes, she was on a rampage! But she never slipped on her professional commitments, and I truly admire her for that. — AMRITA ARORA

MY GRANDMOM'S GOND LADDOOS

Ingredients:

Half cup wholewheat flour

Half cup to 3/4 cup jaggery powder (as sweet as you like it)

Less than half cup gond

3 tbsp desiccated coconut

Cardamom (elaichi) powder to taste

Roughly chopped dried fruits (almonds, cashews, walnuts, etc.)

Ghee for cooking

Method:

Heat a little ghee and fry the chopped dried fruits till they are slightly brown. Add the desiccated coconut and sauté very lightly. Leave aside.

Fry gond in ghee on a low flame. Once fried, cool and blend into small pieces.

Roast the flour in 2–3 tbsp ghee. Once roasted, add the desiccated coconut and dried fruit mixture and cook lightly.

Mix all the ingredients together and roll it into laddoos. This proportion should make 8–10 medium-sized laddoos.

MY PAYA SOUP

Ingredients:

500 gm paya

A little minced ginger, garlic and onion (as per taste)

2 chopped onions

Water, oil, turmeric (haldi) and salt (for cooking)

Method:

Cook the minced ginger, garlic and onion in about 1 tbsp oil for 3 minutes.

Sauté the chopped onions for 3 minutes. Add the paya to it.

Add all of the above to a pressure cooker with one litre water and haldi and salt.

Cook for 20 minutes (that is, 5 minutes on high flame and then 15 minutes on low flame).

The soup is ready to eat. This proportion is for two.

I have worked with Kareena for many years now. She wasn't expecting to get pregnant either time. We didn't plan anything special to get pregnant or improve fertility levels. I just advised her to soak five raisins and two strands of saffron overnight in fresh water and drink the whole concoction in the morning. This is actually great for your periods, PCOD, fertility, etc. She has always been fit, active and food conscious. She went about her life as normal. She worked non-stop throughout both her pregnancies, especially during Covid, and I think she achieved that because she has always been healthy and conscientious. She eats right and, during her pregnancies, she ate right as much as her cravings allowed! Trust me, she loves her cheat foods! Whenever I make the traditional Maharashtrian fried chaklis (called bhajani) at home, I have to send it to her! But she got back into shape in six months post Taimur, and the second time will be no different. I remember she was walking the ramp for a fashion show less than two months after she had Taimur, and she looked amazing. We focus so much on getting the weight off post pregnancy that we forget to focus on the shape we are in before pregnancy and what our lifestyle has been like. The biggest change in both Kareena's and Saif's life over the past ten years is that they have made a conscious effort to go to bed early and that has made a great difference to their health. Barring night shoots and a handful of parties, they have been very good about this. And this has ultimately helped her overall health, stamina, mood, hormonal balance and nutrient sufficiency. Everything that is important for a smooth pregnancy! – RUJUTA DIWEKAR

The four pillars of a healthy pregnancy

I am going to give you a short answer to any long questions you might have about pregnancy nutrition right before we start. You need to be healthy and fit before you conceive your baby. You may or may not be pregnant, but you still need to be well. Our body and our mind is one holistic unit that works on a few common principles: sleep on time, exercise, eat right and drink water. These principles will be especially important for you when you are pregnant. Why?

1. I cannot emphasize enough on sleep. Your body basically goes through an immense ascent and withdrawal of hormones during pregnancy and then immediately after. Good sleep is what helps your body adapt to these hormones. Your body needs sleep to burn fat, to recover, to detox, for muscle repair and just to de-stress (see box 'Pregnancy insomnia? Four ways to help you sleep better'). Don't forget that 20-minute afternoon power nap, if you can squeeze it in.

2. Without exercise and without any stimuli on your bones, joints and muscles, your body is just not primed (or motivated) to absorb the nutrients you're trying to feed it. Exercise also increases your insulin sensitivity and reduces stress.

3. If you're missing good and wholesome food, you're missing a balanced state of digestion and hormones. Mood swings, bloating, acidity, nausea, lethargy and digestive issues are all the by-products (see section 'How to eat right through your pregnancy').

4. The water balance in your body becomes very important during pregnancy as the placenta and amniotic fluid depend on it. You need water to form new tissue, make amniotic fluid, form more blood, to relieve constipation, prevent UTIs, to decrease the risk of swelling and haemorrhoids, to keep your body cool and to manage the flow of all those toxins from your baby and you. It is here that your kidneys kick in – these are the core front-line workers of your pregnancy. It is your kidneys that continuously adjust to the new fluctuating

levels of fluids and electrolytes in your body. All these little fellows want in return is some mindful eating so they can cope better and keep your body in check (blood pressure and acidity included).

Lastly, alongside these basics, a pregnant woman needs to pay attention to all her micronutrients – especially calcium and iron and vitamin B12. How do you work that into your everyday life without driving yourself crazy? Calcium and iron are like love – you will find them in the most unexpected places. A few simple tips? Have millets and nuts. And all your vegetables. Pick up the sabzis that have a local name and are available with your local vegetable vendor. Forget about kale and asparagus!

In short...

Finish dinner by 8.30 p.m., get a proper night's sleep, eat a varied home-cooked meal and have dahi every day (even as chaach or raita). Hydrate, hydrate! Have a lot of water, coconut water, nimbu pani and homemade sherbets (like amla, kokum and so on). Make yoga and/or gym a part of your life. Try and stay active for at least 30 minutes a day or a total of three hours a week. And finally, don't underestimate the power of an afternoon power nap! Keep time for recreation too.

Your essential pregnancy nutrients

Through your pregnancy, you'll read about all the nutrients important for you and the baby. It might make your head a little dizzy! Here are the five essential nutrients your body needs during this time. Remember, eating a balanced home-cooked Indian diet and seasonal and local food will meet most of these needs.

- **Folic acid:** Folic acid is the synthetic (medical) version of folate, and folate is a type of naturally occurring vitamin B. Folic acid is very important – particularly for the first 12 weeks – because it prevents neural tube defects in the baby which affect the spine, spinal cord and brain. Folate-rich foods include all lentils, beetroot, banana, nuts and seeds.

- **Protein:** Protein is the 'builder' of your body; it aides in the development and repair of cells, muscles, tissue and organs, which means it is vital to the growth and development of your baby too. Dals, milk products, eggs, meat and fish, nuts and seeds, and whole grains are good sources of protein.

- **Calcium:** Calcium strengthens your baby's bones, muscles, teeth, heart and nerves. If you're not consuming enough calcium your growing baby will deplete your body's calcium resources, which basically means you're risking bone loss and osteoporosis later in life. Calcium-rich foods include all dairy products, ragi and sesame seeds.

- **Iron:** Your body uses iron to make extra blood for your baby and you. It transfers oxygen to both of you and keeps your RBC count up too. A good RBC count keeps your energy levels up. Fish, meat, eggs, spinach, dried fruits and sesame seeds are all iron rich.

How to eat right through your pregnancy

I have always told Kareena and all my clients that eating should not be complicated. Eat ghar ka khana as much as possible, the food you have grown up with, and keep your meals small. This is especially the case during pregnancy. However, your health will depend on not just the food you eat but also on how well your body absorbs these nutrients. Stress as well as lack of sleep and exercise all contribute to poor assimilation of nutrients. This is why eating right is only one pillar of pregnancy eating. Now with that caveat out of the way, here is a simple meal plan that you can tweak to your taste (see section 'The top three foods per trimester').

This plan ensures you have enough calcium, folic acid and protein in your diet, that your blood sugars are stable and that you are assimilating enough iron. If you can ensure these five things in your eating, most of your basic pregnancy nutritional problems will be dealt with. Your dahi, bedtime milk and chaach will give you protein and calcium. Rice and dals, dosas and peanut chikkis will give you folic acid and also protein. The laddoos, ghee, chikkis and small frequent meals will aid in blood sugar regulation. And your dried fruits and iron karhai preparations will boost iron levels. Your everyday Indian foods contain all the wholesome nutrients you need for a healthy pregnancy within them already. Just eat and enjoy and don't stress yourself by breaking up your food into nutrient groups and overthinking it.

Before breakfast

Wake up to a fresh fruit and some mixed nuts (like almonds, walnuts, cashew) and dried fruits (like raisins, dates, apricots). Nuts and dried fruits complement each other. Dried fruits like raisins are high in iron, while nuts will help you absorb the iron better. Soak your dried fruits the night before.

Breakfast

About an hour to 90 minutes after you wake up, have breakfast. This is when you drink your tea or coffee; try and limit it to a cup. Have a hot, freshly cooked breakfast – idli, dosa, poha, upma, dhokla, porridge, paratha or sheera. Egg and toast is another good combination. You can use a variety of ingredients like ragi, rice, jowar, oats, dalia and millets, but don't mix them up. Remember, one grain at a time.

Mid-morning snack

Have a mid-morning snack of a drink and something to nibble. It will keep you hydrated and energized. Go for coconut water (coconut water taken after 2 p.m. might give you gas, so always have it in the morning), nimbu pani, any of our traditional sherbets such as kokum sherbet, misri jal, aam panna, bel sherbet or kanji. You can also have a laddoo or a piece of peanut chikki, or a handful of peanuts, makhana, etc.

Lunch

Consider any vegetable with roti, bhakri or paratha made of different grains like jowar, bajra, ragi and buckwheat. Stick to one grain at a time. Dal, rice and vegetables or dahi-rice with vegetables is also great. Add a bowl of sprouts and that spoon or two of ghee at lunch. Ghee really helps with the post-lunch energy slump and hunger craving. You can have some dahi too; remember you need a serving of dahi every day.

I would recommend you eat meat or seafood a few times a week; definitely not every day and not for every meal. Also, ideally, it should be a part of a larger meal – say, a chicken or fish curry with a vegetable and roti/rice. This would work better than a simple fillet of grilled fish with some vegetables on the side.

Late afternoon/early evening snack

Don't skip that late afternoon/early evening snack. You can also split this up into two small snacks, at about 3.30 p.m. and then 6 p.m. approximately. At this time, based on how hungry you are and how much energy you need, consider these snack options: (1) fresh seasonal fruit or fresh fruit milkshake, (2) a glass of chaach, (3) a laddoo/chikki made with coconut, jaggery, rajgira, rawa, peanuts, (4) a raab pudding, pej, kanji or dosa made of ragi or bajra, (5) a bowl of poha, khakra or a homemade snack like chivda or mathri and so on, (6) toast with egg, chutney or paneer (7) a simple roti with jaggery. Ideally, do not opt for any caffeinated beverages after this point of time in the day to ensure you have undisturbed sleep at night.

WHY YOU NEED TO DITCH YOUR PROTEIN-ONLY MEALS DURING PREGNANCY

For your body to be able to assimilate protein and to be able to use amino acids properly (which are building blocks for growth, repair, wear and tear and maintenance) you have to ensure you are eating protein with the correct combination of carbs and fats, i.e., as part of a larger meal. Rice and fish curry or egg and toast will allow your body to access and use the amino acids for what they are meant. Your pregnancy is one time you need your carbs to work as carbs and not have your proteins and amino acids being destroyed in the process for energy metabolism. These nutrients must be spared for – and I repeat – growth, repair, wear and tear and maintenance.

Dinner

Dinner should be a light meal, one that is nutritious and easy to digest. Finish no later than 8.30 p.m. so you have plenty of time to digest the food. As your pregnancy progresses, only eat how much you can – as your appetite may also reduce. Try to stick to rice-based dishes and some well-cooked vegetables and your non-vegetarian item, if you eat that. The key to dinner is to eat food that gets easily digested and enables restful sleep. Rice is excellent for this. Dal and rice should be your best friend these nine months. It is calming, comforting, light; a meal that your gut bacteria recognizes and thrives on. If you alternate between rice and roti/bread in the day, make rice your dinner meal. A good dinner can be as simple as khichdi, kanji, dal, rice and vegetables. If you must eat out, pick lunch over dinner. A badly digested dinner can mess with your sleep. And sleep is very important when you're pregnant. Even non-vegetarian options for that matter are best had for lunch.

PREGNANCY INSOMNIA? FOUR WAYS TO HELP YOU SLEEP BETTER

1. Maintain an exercise routine
2. Try and avoid screens for games and social media post dinner and before bed
3. Keep your room and your body as cool as possible
4. Drink a glass of milk with a pinch of nutmeg (jaiphal), a pinch of turmeric (haldi) and three to four soaked cashews before bed. Add a little sugar to this drink if you like. This wonderful nightcap will regulate your hormones, boost immunity and help you with bloating/swelling too

---

Post dinner

I swear by a cup of milk at bedtime for pregnant women. It aids in sleep and gives you that additional dose of calcium and protein.

Finally, I would add the following few suggestions to my checklist for eating right.

Add a chutney or a pickle to your meal: These are quiet little warriors that can aide your gut health, improve insulin response, provide good fats and help assimilate nutrients. The common pregnancy backache and constipation will begin to ease off when your body properly assimilates the fibre and calcium from your food and from your supplements (see box 'Traditional foods to alleviate pregnancy symptoms').

Eat mindfully: Always eat your meals, as they say, 'shanti se' – food can be your pleasure and your joy. Eat without distractions. This way, you will be mindful about when you need to stop! My clients always ask me when to stop eating and how they will know. I always tell them that they should eat such that they feel slightly hungry within two to three hours. For example, after your lunch, you should be able to have a bowl of dahi in the next two to three hours. Also, every time you delay a meal, you will tend to overeat. Keep to your meal times.

Be moderate: People have fears surrounding 'warming' foods and superstitions about 'lactation' foods. To them I'd say, eat as you always did: healthy and nutritious. Whether it's a pineapple, papaya or any sabzi you enjoy – just eat it in the right amounts, i.e., eat till the point you feel light in the stomach. Don't have any food fears. Don't fall for fads. Keep your meals basic, eat seasonal and eat in the right quantities.

Eat seasonal: Eat seasonal fruits, vegetables and grains. Bajra is a great grain for winter as is makki (cornmeal). Jowar is good for the summer. And ragi is great year round (especially in the summer). Keep buckwheat (kuttu) for the days of fasts. Go the extra mile to have mangoes in summer, lychees and plums in monsoon and strawberries and guavas in winter. Pick the local bor, jamun, tinda or suran. Forget about those imported cold storage fruits or vegetables. And eat your fruits and vegetables rather than smooshing them into shakes, juices and smoothies. Chewing your fruits and vegetables is actually great for your oral health too.

Embrace laddoos and chikkis: Things made with dry coconut, sesame seeds, mixed nuts and seeds, peanuts and jaggery bring you nutrients and steady your sugars. Those traditional Indian laddoo ingredients have phytonutrients that are good for your gut, skin, hair and blood sugar.

Avoid packaged foods: Thrilled to find your favourite chips, cookies and chaklis being sold low-sugar, gluten-free, fat-free, baked or made of nachni? Let me tell you the hard truth. They don't work. You're risking extra sodium and sugars with packaged foods. If you cannot completely avoid packaged foods, limit them to a bare minimum. Ready-to-eat meals, boxed Greek yogurt, aerated drinks, cookies, noodles, bottled sauces – these fall under the packaged food umbrella.

Craving fried food, go homemade: If it's homemade chakli, murukku, mathri or even samosas, bhajias or vadas – it's fine. Indulge your craving for that puri or 'nashta' every so often if you feel like. Once in 10–15 days is okay. But do it at home; deep-fried, baked or shallow-fried, as you please. Relish it. If you rarely opt for these treats, just go the whole hog and indulge that craving. Why settle for air-fried and baked versions? Else you'll think it's cool to crave an ice cream at 11 p.m. or you'll want a chocolate at breakfast the next morning. And then you slip down that rabbit hole. This is a habit you need to correct. Don't just pile on the pounds because you're pregnant!

Ghee is your best friend: Have ghee with every meal. Ghee ensures that your blood sugars rise slowly.

Cook in an old-fashioned iron karhai: This helps maintain iron levels in your body, which is crucial in pregnant women.

Dahi every day: If you follow the basic meal plans, your calcium needs will be met. But this is just a reminder yet again about how important that is. Try and have one bowl of dahi/dahi-rice/raita, one glass of chaach/lassi and one glass of bedtime milk.

Incorporate millets in your diet: Have jowar or bajra rotis, ragi porridges or muddes. Try and eat some rajgira (laddoos especially) a few times a week.

PLEASE! I REALLY CAN'T DO ROTI-SABZI EVERY DAY

I know I have largely been talking about sabzis, grains and dahi. And you're wondering what's up with that. Well, I am a devoted Indian food proponent. But it is only normal to want a change of taste! Ideally, you can pick anything based on rice. Rice and millets are great for dinner in pan-Asian, Mexican and Italian flavours. And it will satisfy your craving for that non-Indian meal. Go for it with any curry or vegetable or meat dish. If you plan to crack open that box of white pasta once in a while – that's okay too. But use a fresh home-cooked sauce. My advice – in an ideal scenario – would be to indulge in that one weekly 'cheat meal' properly, but be good for the other six days. Have whatever you want. And please don't skip lunch because you want to have that pasta for dinner. And don't hit the treadmill with a vengeance the morning after an indulgent meal either. When you do indulge, enjoy it guilt free!

Diet-related pregnancy complications

As mentioned before, much of pregnancy eating is really healthy balanced eating at any time of your life. If you have maintained this, and your body has absorbed all the nutrients, you will get everything you need to have a healthy pregnancy. For example, rice–dal–dahi will give you protein and folic acid. However, pregnant women do need three nutrients – calcium, iron and protein – in proper quantities, alongside folic acid. Even if they are eating right, many women aren't also able to assimilate the nutrients at the right level. Your tests and ultrasounds at the doctors may show up anaemia or a foetus that's not growing at the right pace – and you will be asked to up your iron or protein levels respectively. These are extremely common problems. You may also suffer from other pregnancy-related health issues that will require special eating such as gestational diabetes. This is also very common.

Iron and anaemia

The truth is that most pregnant women in India do start their pregnancies with low iron levels, and about 50 per cent of pregnant Indian women suffer from iron deficiency anaemia and low haemoglobin. It has nothing to do with being vegetarian or non-vegetarian. You need 20–30 mg of iron per day during pregnancy.

Almost all pregnant women are given an iron supplement – either from trimester one or the start of trimester two.

Now your haemoglobin levels will go down during pregnancy. Haemoglobin is measured as a concentration. And because your blood volume goes up during pregnancy, your tests record a lower level of haemoglobin too. As long as you're maintaining it above 10–10.5, your ferritin levels aren't crashing, and as long as your B12 levels are good, you don't have to worry about iron or anaemia. Eat well and don't skip meals.

Are you unable to absorb the iron properly? Iron absorption is aided by other nutrients. The big one is vitamin C (nimbu, amla). But so is vitamin A (pumpkin, sweet potato), vitamin B12 (dahi, chaach, kadhi) and different types of nuts and seeds. This is why you should wake up to some dried fruits and nuts every morning. Eat palak, pumpkin, doodhi – all your regular sabzis. Have a good side dose of amla achaar or nimbu achaar with your iron-rich meal or pop your daily iron supplement with a shot of nimbu juice. Try to cook in an iron skillet, and eat from a silver plate. Lack of sleep, minimal exercise, popping antacids, excess caffeine and raw juice (yes, even raw 'iron-rich' spinach juice!) inhibit the optimal assimilation of iron. If you're low on iron, you get low on energy and your nausea tends to get worse.

Protein

Of course pregnant women need more protein. There are no numbers and figures attached to it. But there is a thumb rule – you need to consume your proteins as part of a well-balanced and wholesome meal plan (see box 'Why you need to ditch your protein-only meals during pregnancy'). Dahi, dals and nuts should be part of your daily diet. Don't eat your lentils/sprouts without cooking them or soaking overnight. It is tough to digest. Ease up on your gut during pregnancy as your digestion does take a bit of a beating. Remember, eat foods you recognize. Don't rush into eating too much lentils at a time just because you've heard it is protein rich. Combine your proteins with roti or rice, so your body receives both essential and non-essential amino acids.

Help! I need to up my protein in three weeks!

Well, a wholesome and diverse diet with fresh, seasonal and local produce; eating frequent meals; staying physically active and sleeping on time – all of that allows for better protein assimilation and protein synthesis in your body. Your proteins are best consumed with the correct combination of carbs and fats, i.e., as part of a larger meal. And when it comes to whey protein shakes – it is not a good idea to start a shake now. If you have been using protein shakes before you got pregnant, you can continue them if you like. Add the following to your daily diet if you need a boost: dahi, chaach, khichdi, sprouts (soaked overnight and then sprouted). You can add egg and fish/chicken to your diet every day but remember to do so as part of the full meal. And, as I have said, don't underestimate sleep and exercise – you're pregnant, not sick, so stay active. Exercise is a great protein preserver. But remember, food isn't a magic pill that will give you instant results – a sustained balanced diet, keeping all the fundamentals in mind, is your best path.

Calcium

Women need significantly more calcium during pregnancy – about 1000 mg per day. You'll need this nutrient to build the baby's bones and teeth. Women can become extremely depleted of calcium by the end of their pregnancies. With inadequate calcium, you may feel weak and lose bone strength, which in turn means you may take longer to get back in shape post pregnancy. If you have your dahi/chaach/milk every day alongside your balanced diet (you should be adding millets and nuts to your diet), your calcium needs will be met. Your doctor will probably also give you a calcium supplement, to be on the safe side, which you will need to continue with post pregnancy. Vitamin D is a great buddy of calcium and helps it to absorb better. If you're low on vitamin D, your doctor may prescribe a supplement. But a daily dose of sunlight and an afternoon nap also help with vitamin D assimilation.

I AM LACTOSE INTOLERANT! HOW DO I GET ENOUGH CALCIUM?

Keep it simple! Rajgira in the form of laddoos or chikkis, ragi in the form of dosas or mudde, a good handful of nuts and a great mix of fresh local vegetables can help you meet your requirements. Don't switch to nut milks (almond, soy, oat, etc.) to compensate for regular milk.

Gestational diabetes

Women who have gestational diabetes don't really need to eat anything different and specific. However, I would add this: avoid all packaged and processed foods, including packaged cereals. Skip juices; instead eat fruits. Have home-cooked meals as far as possible and keep it simple: roti, sabzi, dal, chaawal. Avoid restaurant food and takeouts. Try not to eat out more than once a week.

The top three foods per trimester

There is now an infobesity (overload of information) on every trimester: the hormones, the foetus, nutrients needed and everything. In spite of this, information on what to eat in the Indian context is non-existent. And though hormones and foetal growth will follow a universal pattern, the food part needs to be localized. The lost wisdom needs to be unearthed from our kitchens, translated from the vernacular to a language that resonates with nutrition science and, more importantly, be allowed to support the working woman, both nutritionally and emotionally, in this phase.

So, in every trimester, I am going to list out the three most important foods that you must incorporate into your plan.

Traditional foods to alleviate pregnancy symptoms

1. Gulkand (a traditional preserve made of rose petals, khaddi shakkar and cardamom) with water helps in nausea and constipation
2. Add ginger and lemongrass to that cup of chai – if you feel acidic
3. A simple panchamrit (honey, milk, dahi, sugar, ghee and saffron) keeps your hormones balanced

4. A pinch of hingashtak (a digestive powder made with shunthi, sonth, kali miri, saindha namak, pippali, hing, ajwain and jeera) is good for gut bacteria. Hing is the main ingredient, and the rest is according to your taste and tolerance

The top three foods for T1

The first trimester is easily the most challenging and critical part of your pregnancy, and though the baby will grow on autopilot from here on, there are some foods which will help you go through this phase smoothly.

1. Hing or asafoetida

A common Indian herb or spice that has antibacterial, antiviral properties and is a digestive aid. It's the one spice that will help keep the nausea and bloating down, stoke your appetite and help you eat better. Most of us use it in tadkas, especially for dals, and it aids absorption of nutrients from the dal. It also plays an important role in helping to improve our mood, and relieves the fatigue or drowsiness that sometimes accompany T1.

How to use it:
- Pinch of hing in chaas along with kalanamak to keep the acidity down
- In tadkas for dals and sabzis
- Add a pinch in coconut oil and massage on the tummy for relief from gas and bloating

2. Ragi/Nachni/Mandua or finger millet

Ragi is a nutrient-rich food and it provides us everything that we need in this crucial phase – from amino acids to calcium, iron to fibre. It regulates our appetite and prevents overeating, is very easy to both cook and digest, and even keeps a check on the lipid levels (triglycerides – the circulating fat in the bloodstream, high levels of which will make you prone to diabetes). Also, long term, it is required for good lactation too, so it's good to start including it in your meals, at least a couple of days a week from now.

How to use it:
- Can make bhakris or rotis with it, and while it takes some practice, the ragi dosa is easy to make and delicious. Just dosa and chutney also make for a light meal when you do not feel like eating a full meal or roti–sabzi–dal.
- Sprouted ragi is even better and can be stored/refrigerated for a week. Can turn into a quick breakfast meal – malt/satva or kanji or ambil – and you can teach your husband to cook this.
- Ragi laddoo is made by rolling it with sesame, almonds, peanuts and coconut.

3. Beets

These are rich in phytonutrients, called betalains, and are known for their antioxidant, detoxifying and anti-inflammatory properties. And though beetroot is not a good source of iron (its leaves are), it's an excellent source of folic acid. It also contains high amounts of manganese, magnesium and copper and even vitamins like B6 and C. The nutrition profile is good for nerve support, prevents calf pain and varicose veins too. If you can get your hands on beet leaves, eat them too by cooking them like a palak or spinach bhaji; it's a good source of iron and other minerals.

How to use it:
- Simply pressure- or steam-cook it and eat a beetroot as a part of a meal or a mid-meal by itself.
- Beet poriyal is an excellent and nutrient-rich sabzi that's easy to cook.
- Add pieces of beetroot to rice or khichdi – easiest way to cook and eat.

The top three foods for T2

Though this is officially the easiest time of the pregnancy, this is also the period that is going to decide how smooth your delivery is and how quickly you get back in shape post it. And without the support of essential fatty acids and the fat soluble vitamins that come with them, vitamins A, D, E and K, changes to the skin and hair can occur too. So T2 is actually nature's way to give you the time to have everything in your control before any damage – stretch marks, loss of hair, pigmentation, etc. – can take place. And to do this job are nature's very own beauty pills – the ones that keep blood sugars under control, help improve bone and joint health and provide the amino acids that keep the skin supple and fresh. Here we go:

1. Nutmeg or jaiphal
This spice is used in tiny amounts to flavour kheer, halwas and laddoos. Rich in antioxidant properties and minerals, jaiphal is used to improve digestion, prevent hair loss and fine lines or wrinkling of the skin, and to reduce blood pressure. The key

though, as with any spice, is to use it intelligently, that is, in amounts that are tiny enough to just hint at the presence of the spice. Because it is exactly in these amounts that it is medicinal. It even helps in the production of red blood cells and keeps fatigue away, which many of you will feel through your pregnancy.

How to use it:
- Flavouring agent in laddoos, kheer, halwa.
- Mix with besan and milk, apply to skin to help achieve a smooth texture and prevent itching (especially for itchy nipples or thighs).
- Add a pinch to milk and have it at bedtime for better sleep.

2. Ghee

Ah! You were waiting for this one. From the short chain fatty acids that help the intestines function better and support the growth of good bacteria to helping accelerate fat burning and making food delicious, ghee is truly the most divine fat on earth. Its benefits are many; one of the most important ones during pregnancy is that the addition of ghee to food slows down the rate at which blood sugars climb, and this quality really helps support both the thyroid and the insulin hormone. The key here is to make it from full fat milk from indigenous (desi) cows, and if not desi cows, then buffaloes, but never Jersey or Holstein cows. Make it at home, and if not home, buy from a trustworthy, small gaushala.

How to use it:
- Add a teaspoon or two to your rotis and rice. If there is a history of diabetes in the family, add a little extra, as the addition of essential fat helps support the insulin function.

- You can use it for tadka or cooking of dals, sabzis and biryanis. And of course in laddoos, halwa and barfis.
- Rub the soles of your feet with ghee in the night to prevent constipation and induce better sleep.

3. Foxtail millet/Kangani/Tenai/Rala/Koralu

Since millets grow across India, you will have local names based on the region you come from. The foxtail millet looks like couscous or tiny grains of rice or rava and is cooked exactly the way you would make rice. From upma to pulao to kheer, it blends superbly in all regional recipes. It tastes especially nice when made with peanuts or cooked like plain rice and eaten with lentils. It is known to reduce blood sugars and c-reactive protein (something that rises when inflammation or BP rises), and, like all millets, helps improve the HDL levels (important for a healthy heart).

How to use it:
- Cook like rice and eat with lentils or dals.
- Can be sprouted and made into malt/porridge, which makes vitamin B more available. Or make it like a kheer with dry fruits.
- Make it like a dalia or upma with veggies and peas.

The top three foods for T3

T3 can be a tiring phase and a test of patience, literally. On the one hand you want to let it all go, on the other you are constantly aware that once you do let go, nothing will ever be the same again. The baby will change your life forever, and other than her health, security and well-being, nothing else will matter. The next six months can be quite overwhelming. So behenon, to keep the mind calm and the body strong, here are the foods for this phase.

1. Turmeric/Haldi

The West has discovered it too, the active curcumin compound in haldi has the ability to stop the degeneration of both brain and muscle, and its antioxidant properties are the stuff that patent battles are made of. Turmeric in India is consumed both tender and mature, and remains extremely useful in all its forms. It is also used for its ability to prevent eye strain, protect the heart, nerves and what have you, so don't miss out on this – but don't have it in capsule form. It works best when it's part of a wholesome diet, so let's not turn into people who eat raw salads and pop turmeric pills. It's especially useful during pregnancy as it's also an antidepressant – this is a time when your emotions will be stirred, and you may feel vulnerable and fragile.

How to use it:
- In tadkas for dal/sabzis/khichdi. Follow the pattern taught at home about when exactly to add it while cooking.
- Tender turmeric – make a pickle or add in chai with lemongrass, ginger and honey.
- Add a pinch of turmeric to chana or masoor dal paste, mix it with milk and use it while bathing; especially useful to prevent pigmentation and lines post pregnancy.

2. Moong dal

Amongst all the lentils, the most satvik bean is moong. It remains the most precious dal in the eyes of our grandmoms for its easy digestibility, dense nutritional profile – folic acid, vitamin B6, minerals, proteins, etc. – and for its neutral taste. Moong dal is the least gas forming of all dals, a good quality to have if you are an expectant mother. Moreover, it helps you to accelerate fat burning, and reduces the risk of all degenerative diseases, including diabetes, BP and cancer.

How to use it:
- Once they have been soaked overnight and sprouted, you can cook them well for maximum nutrient absorption.
- Make dal or khichdi out of it.
- Make chatpata items like chivda or chilla out of it to kill the boredom of eating bland food and without the risk of eating junk.

3. Rice

Rice and dal is one of the world's most complete foods nutritionally and also what's most soothing to your stomach. As you near D-Day, and are feeling exhausted, nervous and low on appetite, lean into this miraculous food for nutrition, easy digestion and comfort.

How to use it:
- Cook rice and eat with dals/lentils/kadhi/dahi/milk.
- Make pej or kanji – a light soup that retains the vitamin B of rice and is light to digest.
- Give a tadka or chonkha to last night's leftover rice to turn into a quick and delicious breakfast meal.

Excerpted and adapted with permission from *Pregnancy Notes: Before, During and After* **by Rujuta Diwekar, published by Westland Publications Limited, 2017**

THE POWER OF ALIV

This is my post-pregnancy superfood. Aliv laddoos are an integral part of traditional Indian post-pregnancy foods. Note that it's a post-delivery food, not something to take during pregnancy.

What is aliv? These are scarlet coloured seeds, also known as halim or garden cress seeds. It is a source of essential fatty acids, like linoleic and arachidic, and has iron, amino acids and phytonutrients.

What are the benefits of aliv? Your body will be in a hormonal churn post delivery – aliv helps hair and skin health. It can keep postpartum depression at bay and help you absorb micronutrients like folic acid and minerals like iron and calcium.

How to eat aliv? Traditionally, Indian grandmothers would soak aliv seeds in coconut water and then cook them with grated coconut, ghee and jaggery and roll them into bright red laddoos. When aliv is mixed with coconut and ghee, you get the perfect ratio of omega 3, 6, 9. Alternatively, aliv seeds soaked overnight can be turned into kheer or added to a cup of milk and consumed. Now, what if you don't want to eat those laddoos? Try the garden cress plant's baby greens as a garnish on your food or turn it into a chutney.

Adapted with permission from *Indian Superfoods* by Rujuta Diwekar, published by Juggernaut Books, 2016

What should I avoid during pregnancy

Play it safe when you're pregnant. Don't introduce any foreign (i.e., new) foods into your diet – by that I mean foods you haven't eaten before. You don't know if it will sit well in your stomach. Eat from restaurants you are already familiar with. Don't try out new places. Better safe than sorry! There are no hard no-nos in my books (except alcohol and smoking). If you've had seafood, milk and milk products all your life, it is safe for you to continue doing so unless you develop sudden intolerance.

If you're a vegetarian, please don't think you now have to start eating an egg to get more protein. An eggetarian needn't start eating meat. And if you eat meat, you don't have to give it up. Remember that the foods you ate got you pregnant in the first place. So continue with the same food traditions. To sum it up, don't make major alterations to your pre-existing (healthy!) food choices.

Caffeine

You can have a cup – and maximum two – of tea or coffee a day. And enjoy your tea/coffee with sugar. This is basically the global recommendation of 200 mg (maximum 300 mg) per day. Be mindful about overdosing. There are many indirect sources of caffeine entering your bloodstream – through soft drinks, dark chocolate, desserts and some herbal teas. Any tea made of actual tea leaves – whether black, green, oolong or white – will add caffeine to your cup. Chamomile, mint, tulsi or peppermint tea, for instance, will not have caffeine. And remember, no coffee and tea on an empty stomach. Have it with your breakfast.

Alcohol

I tell all my clients to completely avoid alcohol through pregnancy.

Seafood

Continue having the fish you always had.

9

FITNESS
With Namrata Purohit

My body

I have to admit I got fat during both my pregnancies. I put on 25 kg at Taimur's time and 19 kg with Jeh. (I made myself happy with the 2 or 3 kg I lost on the OT table once my boys were born!) I would look at pictures of pregnant Hollywood celebrities and wonder how they were so skinny. They seemed to only put on weight on their belly! I am not like that. But I am proud of the way in which I carried both my pregnancies.

I was fit and healthy through my pregnancies – I could work and stay on my feet pretty much non-stop. But I didn't follow a very elaborate exercise routine while I was pregnant. Maybe I should have! Exercising through your pregnancy is not only good for you and your baby, it helps to keep up your strength post delivery too. I was active, though. I walked a lot. Even during the lockdown I would meet a friend every evening and walk with her in my building compound or hers.

But I didn't do much more. I stopped training at the gym and lifting weights the moment I realized I was pregnant with Taimur. There was no reason for it. I just did! I walked every day and did a few months of light yoga till my second trimester. That was it. I was too busy enjoying my pregnancy and indulging in all my favourite foods. It was one big party.

When I was pregnant with Jeh, we were locked down in any case. I was also much lower on energy than I was during my first. I was just grateful I could find the strength to fulfil my professional commitments, otherwise I would have been completely cut up. During my second pregnancy, I just about managed to catch an evening walk whenever I could and I did a couple of months of yoga online. But let me be frank, the yoga was pretty half-hearted. I was dedicated to my Kegels, though. I did at least 60 counts every evening before I went to bed.

Usually, I work out diligently. And I work out hard! I am also absolutely devoted to yoga. I love it; it centres me. I got back into shape in less than a year after I had Taimur. In fact, I was pretty much back on track in six months, though for a fleeting moment after I had Taimur I wondered if I'd ever get my old body back. But I had to take it on like a boss girl – and I am pretty confident I will after Jeh too!

I resumed work soon after Taimur was born and I will after Jeh too. I still have the same instinct as I did before: to bring my life back on track within a year, to get back on set, to exercise and diet and juggle life with two children. Given the pandemic and the lockdown situation, things are slower this time. After the first few days post delivery, I simply started by walking around in my house terrace – just about 30 minutes or so. Two months after delivery, I continued walking or using the treadmill at home, trying to stay active and counting my steps. However, I can sense my hormones are taking longer to normalize this time around. For a good two to three months post Jeh, I was exhausted. With Taimur, I was back at the gym in a little over a month.

But I have the motivation and the energy to reclaim my life, calm my baby, get everything in order and be back on my feet. Millions of women across the world have done it. And I am no different. Can I pull it off? I did it once and I will do it again!

Kareena is one of my favourite people to work with: she's fun, loving and a total blast! Let me tell you right away that she decided not to work out during her pregnancy and to take it really easy. I think she felt like this was the one time in her life she could completely let go and simply enjoy herself – and, in a way, take advantage of being pregnant. I think there is nothing wrong in that! I think it is really important to listen to your body and do what is comfortable for you. I would always recommend working out, but sometimes it is also okay to do what you want for yourself. What was great was that right after she delivered Taimur, she got back on track, achieving her fitness goals and working extremely hard again. Things were understandably slower post Jeh because of the lockdown and pandemic stress.

If I remember correctly, Kareena jumped on to the Pilates bandwagon and kick-started her fitness journey pretty much a month after she delivered Taimur. In six months, she had lost all the excess weight she had put on during pregnancy and was not only looking but also feeling fit. She worked out four to five days a week, doing Pilates regularly and some amount of cardio exercises too. She is a very diligent and very hard-working student. She never missed her workout and always gave her 100 per cent.

I remember she once asked me for the famous 'Pilates Girl' top from our studio. And I, a little bluntly, told her, 'You have to earn it.' And that was it! She was determined to work on it and earn that top! I still remember the smile on her face and the eyes that said, watch me now! It was incredible! And, sure enough, just a few weeks in, she earned her Pilates Girl top. – NAMRATA PUROHIT

Baby, let's move!

Pregnancy may seem like the quintessential time to sit back and relax, but unless there are complications, it's a good idea to move and exercise to stay in shape and also prevent unnecessary pain. Maintaining a good exercise programme during pregnancy can help you stay healthy and feel your best.

Let's take a look at what exercising during pregnancy can do for you.

- It can reduce back pain caused by increased body weight and the shift in your centre. How? By strengthening the necessary muscles to compensate for the shift in centre.
- It is also said that working out during pregnancy can help prevent constipation and bloating.
- We know this already, but exercising during this phase can help improve your mood.
- It also improves posture, which helps relieve unnecessary pain or discomfort.
- It can help reduce fatigue.
- There is also evidence that working out during pregnancy can help prevent gestational diabetes.

- It will also help prevent excess weight gain, and keep your muscles toned and strong.
- It can help you sleep better, and who doesn't want some good hours of sleep?
- Exercising through your pregnancy can also improve stamina that might be needed during labour and delivery.
- It helps with postpartum recovery.

As you can see, working out during pregnancy offers a lot of benefits. If you have exercised regularly, you should continue. If you haven't exercised, this is a great time to start! However, before you lace up those sneakers and get on the track, ensure that you stop by your doctor and get the green light. Your workouts should also be supervised by a trainer with experience in pre- and postnatal workouts.

Most exercises are safe to do during pregnancy as long as you listen to your body, exercise with caution and do not overdo it. Exercises that are particularly good are those with low impact on the body: like Pilates, yoga, low-impact aerobics, swimming and brisk walks. These activities carry a low chance of injury, benefit the entire body and can be done until the very last day of pregnancy.

If you are an experienced athlete, runner or racquet sports player, you should be able to continue these activities for at least a few months into your pregnancy. But do check in with your doctor. If you have been exercising regularly before you got pregnant, you can most likely continue the same regimen with a few modifications. However, if you are new to exercise, it is advisable to start slow and do exercises that are less complicated and are easy to understand and perform. In essence, continue with what you have been doing; don't do anything new. If you are completely new to exercise, stick to low-impact workouts like walking or yoga (supervised) and build this up incrementally.

It is best to eat at least an hour before you begin exercising and keep drinking enough water throughout.

Pregnancy brings with it a lot of questions, but don't worry, you are not the only one asking them. Let's discuss some of the most frequently asked questions related to exercise and pregnancy.

How much should I do?

How much you exercise during pregnancy depends on how active you have been before getting pregnant and on any health issues you may have. Trying to be active every day can be beneficial and even small things like walking to the kitchen, doing basic household work or walking to your local grocery store can make a difference.

Pregnant women should get at least 150 minutes of moderate intensity exercise every week. This means doing exercises that up the heart rate a bit and get you moving, maybe even breaking into a sweat! You can achieve this by exercising five days a week for 30 minutes at a time or even break it up and do 10 minutes three times through the day. Ideally, it is good to work out for 30 minutes a day, even if you don't do it all at once.

If you have been active you already know your body's capabilities. If you are new to exercising, start slow and don't rush into it. If you want to do the basics at home, take 'baby steps'. For example, you can do a 15-minute walk three times a week to begin with, and then increase it to four and then maybe up the time from 15 to 20 minutes. Basically, opt for gradual progress until you can eventually achieve the 30-minute target, four to five times a week.

CAN I DO HOUSEHOLD CHORES?

Yes. You can do all household chores like you usually would. You might need to slow down a bit as the months go by, but everything is doable and, in fact, it might be a great way to stay active. While it may be ideal that you don't try and stand on narrow surfaces to clean things that are placed high (since your balance may be off) or try and shift a heavy sofa to clean under it, sweeping, vacuuming or mopping are otherwise considered low-impact exercises. When it comes to bending, it isn't your baby that is at risk; it is your discomfort level. Be mindful about bending from your knees (rather than from your waist) and not jerking your back.

What should I avoid?

There are a few activities that could cause harm to you or your baby, and therefore it is recommended you avoid them.

These include contact sports like football and hockey, as there is a possibility of your bump being hit. Activities that have a higher risk of a fall should also be avoided during this time, like skiing, gymnastics and rock climbing. You could also switch from outdoor cycling to indoor cycling just for the added element of safety, as your centre of gravity shifts, and getting used to the new sense of balance might take some time.

If you live in a high-altitude place, you're fine. But avoid exercising at high altitudes otherwise, as your body is already dealing with reduced oxygen levels and exercising would increase the demand on the body. It may result in decreased oxygen supply to you and your baby.

In general, it is also good to avoid classes that are not pregnancy specific as the classes wouldn't be customized or cater to your needs. Make sure you inform the trainer, so that they can customize or modify the routine to suit your needs. It is also recommended to avoid lying on your back for a long period of time, especially after 16 weeks of pregnancy.

How will my changing body affect my exercise regimen?

The biggest and most obvious change is a shift in the centre of gravity because of your growing bump. Due to the shift, your balance might feel different and the chances of falling become greater. It is therefore important to focus on exercises that help keep the body stable and to avoid any exercises that demand a lot of balance, especially if not practised before.

Your joints become more mobile during pregnancy, and that in turn causes the ligaments to become more relaxed. This could make you more susceptible to injury. Hence it is important to take care of your joints and avoid jerky or high impact movements. This means saying no to any exercise where both your feet are off the ground at the same time – like jumping, high knees, burpees, surya namaskars where you jump into your planks. And being mindful about bending from your waist and not getting up too quickly (where your body jerks) or lifting weights too fast.

The need for oxygen also increases in your body. You may also get short of breath more easily as the increase in belly size and the uterus puts more pressure on the diaphragm. Strenuous exercise might become harder over time. The best thing to do is to listen to your body, be aware of its capabilities and also be conscious of how you feel. This way, you are most likely to enjoy your workout and reap its benefits without overexerting yourself. You will know you are overexerting yourself if you can feel your heart racing (or you feel flutters in your chest), you're trying to catch a breath (or you're actively panting), you're feeling too hot and sweaty, or you feel like you're just too exhausted.

What precautions should I take while exercising?

- Stay well hydrated. Drink plenty of water before, during and after exercising
- Avoid lying down on your back
- Avoid standing still for long periods
- Wear the right gear. Wear gear that supports the body. It is important to avoid unnecessary aches and pains. The right sports bra to support your breasts as well as bellyband support later in your pregnancy will help relieve unnecessary stress
- Avoid getting overheated
- Avoid getting breathless. You should be able to talk through all your exercise. If you feel you can't talk, you might be pushing yourself too hard.

How to exercise trimester by trimester (if you have exercised before)

If you have exercised before, what are the modifications you should be making to your routine? Let's look at this, trimester by trimester.

Trimester one

In the first trimester, as long as you are not considered a high-risk pregnancy, you can continue your regular workout routine; just avoid contact sports where you could get hit or sports that have a higher likelihood of a fall. It is also a good idea to start working on your pelvic floor muscles, and improve your core strength and spinal mobility to make the pregnancy easier and prepare you for childbirth. So add these to your routine. For instance, simple things like hip rolls, side planks, planks and side leg raises. However, as stated earlier, if you are new to exercise, start slowly and build up.

Trimester two

In the second trimester, your bump will be growing, and you may want to avoid any high impact activity and exercises that have you lying on the back. Work on stability and strength. Ensure that you keep working on mobility as well as core strength. So, focus on the inner thighs and glutes. Your growing bump adds more pressure on the lower back and pelvis, therefore working on strengthening this area is crucial. Also, do not forget to work the arms, triceps, biceps and chest as you will need these as well in the months to come.

Trimester three

Continue the activity of the second trimester, but it might just need a few modifications. The modification would depend on the exercise you are modifying. For example, for the side lying leg raises, you might want to do standing side leg raises instead, depending on how you feel, how your belly feels and how lying down feels. Keep up the cardiovascular endurance with exercises like walking, swimming, cycling, jogging or dancing. But don't overdo it. And keep focusing on mobility and abdominal strength. Gentle stretches are also great to relieve aches and pains.

What can I or can't I do?

Let's take these FAQs:

Can I go on a hike? Can I climb slopes? Can I take the stairs?
Of course you can do all of these. If you have been hiking in the past and if you are used to climbing slopes, it will probably be safe to continue doing so, even during your pregnancy. It is, however, advisable to stick to more even terrain and to be with someone qualified during these sessions. At the risk of repeating myself, let me reiterate: don't attempt something too new at this time. And always remember to get a go-ahead from your doctor. Take the stairs when you can. But make sure you're comfortable with it and that you have figured out your balance. In an ideal scenario, pace it out – slow and steady steps are best; don't rush up or down the stairs at any point of time.

Should I swim?
If you have been swimming before your pregnancy, you can safely continue to do so. Just have a quick consultation with your doctor to make sure you're not a high-risk pregnancy. Swimming is actually a great non-load-bearing aerobic exercise for your body, which helps with circulation and muscle tone. It gives you a good cardiovascular workout without stressing your spine or joints. The best part? It keeps you cool! Do ensure you check if

the pool you're using is not over chlorinated. Drink some water before and after your swim and do a few simple stretches before you ease into the pool.

Can I do a headstand in trimester three?

It is usually safe to perform most activities and exercises that you did before you got pregnant throughout your pregnancy. You can perform a headstand as long as you did it before and are still comfortable with it, and if you feel good in this position. However, this too must be taken on a case-by-case basis. I would not recommend trying headstands if you have never done it before. Also, it is important to remember that there is a shift in the centre of gravity in your body as your pregnancy progresses, so your balance might be a bit off. It is therefore absolutely inadvisable to perform a headstand without (a) someone around you who can grab your legs when needed; (b) propping yourself against a wall for added safety.

Can I run on a treadmill in trimester one?

The simple answer is yes, you can. However, every person is different, and every pregnancy is different, hence you must consult your doctor and also a personal trainer who can understand your needs. Generally it is safe to walk or even run on the treadmill depending on prior experience as well. Walking is a safer option than running. However, if you used to run before, you can still continue to run during pregnancy. The speed at which you walk or run on the treadmill needs to be determined based on your comfort level and/or under the instructions of a qualified trainer.

I am an HIIT kind of girl: how much can I achieve during pregnancy?

You can practise your high intensity interval training (HIIT) workout safely, like you normally would, especially in the first three months of your pregnancy. But only as long as this is something you have already been accustomed to. It is important to listen to your body and not overstress or push yourself during this stage.

Can I safely lift weights while pregnant?

There is no defined 'safe limit' for pregnant women and weights, so there are no particular guidelines on how much is safe to lift and for how long. Do note at this point of time that how much weight you can lift has more to do with how much you did before you got pregnant, your fitness levels and in general how you are feeling. Even if you have been lifting weights regularly at the gym all your adult life, you may still feel the need to stop lifting weights or reduce your weights as your pregnancy progresses. It is extremely important to be in touch with the doctor. And definitely work with a trainer who has worked with pregnant women or is confident about guiding you through your prenatal fitness routines. You can pretty much do anything you were doing before your pregnancy, as long as your body feels good and feels up to it.

When is it time to stop exercising?

If there are no complications in your pregnancy, you can exercise till the very last day of your pregnancy. Having said that, your body will signal if it feels like it is time to stop exercising. In that case, even on a day-to-day basis, listen to your body and throw in the towel.

Here are the red flags:
- Bleeding from the vagina
- Becoming dizzy or feeling faint
- Any swelling in the body
- Irregular or rapid heartbeat
- Headaches or chest pain
- Feeling shortness of breath even before performing any exercise

In case of any of the above or anything that does not seem normal, consult your doctor and take necessary precautions. Only resume exercising if the doctor permits and keep monitoring your body closely

What are Kegel exercises and how do I perform them?

Kegel exercises can help work and strengthen the pelvic floor muscles. During pregnancy and childbirth, these muscles stretch, but doing Kegel exercises can make the muscles in your pelvis and vaginal area strong.

So, where are these pelvic floor muscles and how do you find them? In Pilates, I teach this as part of core engagement exercises. In order to find your Kegel/pelvic floor muscles, imagine you are in the loo, peeing, and I or anybody for that matter walks in. You stop peeing (or at least hopefully you do); the muscles you use to stop peeing are your pelvic floor muscles. Please don't stop your pee regularly, just do it to find where the muscles are. Now that you know where they are, you know how to engage them. You can practise pulling up the pelvic floor muscles multiple times a day.

Once you know where these muscles are, start by contracting them, hold for a few seconds and then release. The release is as important as the contraction. You can do this for a few minutes three to four times a day. As you start developing strength you can hold the contraction for longer, say, 10–15 seconds, and then release.

This can be done even before you are pregnant and post pregnancy too. Ensuring your pelvic floor muscles are strong can have long-term health benefits.

How soon can I exercise after delivery?

After your delivery, you can work out as soon as you get the go-ahead from your doctor. If you have had an uncomplicated delivery, you can work out as soon as even a few days post birth.

DIASTASIS RECTI

A lot of women experience a split in their abdominal wall muscles during pregnancy. This can most often be reversed post delivery with core strengthening exercises. Simply put, diastasis recti is the gap between your right and left abdominal wall muscles; it is commonly referred to as 'ab separation' or the 'mommy tummy pooch'. It may be a partial or complete separation of the rectus abdominis. It is extremely common during pregnancy as the abdominal wall stretches to accommodate the baby. This may not be very noticeable during pregnancy. But, post delivery, how do you figure out whether you have ab separation? Here are a few signs: (1) you have a back pain or notice a pelvic floor dysfunction (like pelvic muscle spasms, lower back pain, pelvic organ prolapse, hernia, constipation, pain during sexual intercourse, urinary issues); (2) your tummy bulges out a lot more after food, your belly button pops or your tummy bulges/domes out noticeably when you try to sit up after lying down; (3) in an acute case, you can sense your abdominal organs since these are protruding through the muscle gap; (4) lie down on your back with your feet on the floor (i.e., knees bent) and press your fingers (facing downwards) properly above your belly button while raising your neck and shoulders off the floor at the same time. You will very likely sense the clench of your abdominal muscles on your fingers, and you will feel the gap. Right after your delivery, the gap might be the largest. It may take a few weeks to a few months to come back to normal. During this phase, it is advisable not to do any heavy lifting or intense abdominal exercises that might make the gap worse (like crunches). Most of the time, diastasis recti corrects itself after pregnancy, once the abdominal muscles gain strength. If you still experience a large gap three months post pregnancy, specific exercises might help to close the gap. Always train with a qualified professional who understands and can customize the routine for you. It usually involves your pelvic floor muscles and deep abdominal muscle engagement.

Exercises to add to your workout

Finally, let me take you through a series of five exercises that you can add to your general workout routine every trimester, after getting the go-ahead from your doctor of course. It is ideal to get a customized routine from a qualified prenatal expert or qualified prenatal fitness trainer. Every pregnancy is different. But these few exercises can usually be performed in each trimester. These exercises have been suggested as they target the muscles you need to work on through each trimester and also during labour and delivery. They go from working on the inner thighs and lower back to then working on shoulders and triceps in order to be able to hold the baby for longer hours.

Almost all these exercises can be done in each trimester, though some of these exercises may just need some modifications as the months go along. The number of repetitions given here are just a ballpark figure; do modify them as per your comfort level. You can easily do more repetitions than what is suggested here, if you're comfortable. You can do trimester three exercises in trimester one and vice versa; it all depends on how your body is feeling. Remember, these are just a few exercises and not an entire routine. So, you must add more exercises to your routine if you can. It is very important to get cleared by your doctor and to also listen to your body. Before attempting any exercise routine, make sure you are comfortable and confident.

The exercises listed below can be done even if you have never exercised before. However, keep these tips in mind: (1) go slow and steady; (2) do have someone who can watch your form; (3) please get the green light from your doctor.

First trimester

1. Hip rolls

Starting position: Lie down on a mat. Keep your feet flat on the floor and your knees bent. Feet are hip-distance apart. Rest the arms alongside the body.

How to: Inhale to prepare yourself. Exhale. Starting with the tailbone, pick your spine off the mat until your weight rests on your thoracic (upper) spine. Breathe in to maintain the position. Exhale and lower your spine back on the mat and into the neutral spine (i.e., flat spine) position. Repeat this five to eight times. After the last repetition, stay up in the position and do mini pulses, i.e., a very small movement lifting your pelvis up and down.

What are you working: Your abs, obliques and muscles beneath the obliques – the transverse abdominis – as well as the glutes, back (specifically, the multifidus muscles) and shoulder blades.

Keep in mind: Do not rock your pelvis. Make sure you are articulating your spine (i.e., rolling up slowly, one vertebra at a time – the classic Pilates roll-up) while rolling up and down. Do not overextend or hyperextend the back.

2. Push-ups

Starting position: Set your hands slightly more than shoulder-width apart. Feet can be shoulder-width apart or closer together. Generally speaking, the wider apart your feet, the more stable you'll be for your push-ups. Starting with your elbows straight but not locked. Your body should be in a straight line from head to heels. Keep your glutes and core engaged.

How to: Inhale. Steadily lower yourself until your elbows are at a 90-degree angle or less (this depends on your level of experience). Try not to let the elbows go flying out; keep them relatively close to your body. Once you reach the lowest you can go, hold it for a second and then exhale to press back up into the starting position. Do this 15–20 times.

Modification: You can start with a wall push-up, or with your knees down, rather than being in a full palm plank position.

What are you working: The chest muscles (pectorals), deltoids, triceps, abdominals, serratus anterior and even the back and gluteus.

Keep in mind: The whole body should lower as one. Do not leave the gluteus up while doing push-ups. It is not important to go fast. Slow, controlled moves will be more beneficial.

3. Sumo squats

Starting position: Stand with your feet about shoulder-distance apart. The feet should be turned out (laterally rotated from the hip) and back straight. Keep your core engaged and arms relaxed by your side or in front of your chest together.

How to: Inhale to lower yourself down towards the ground, keep your back straight and ensure your knees are right over your ankles. Exhale, engage your glutes, press into your feet and slowly come back up to the starting position. Do this 15–20 times.

What are you working: The glutes, hamstrings, quadriceps and inner thighs.

Keep in mind: Don't let your knees fall inwards while doing the sumo squat; keep them over the ankle and turned outwards. Try not to lean forward, your back should be neutral and straight.

4. Squat and curl

Starting position: Start by standing with your feet parallel and hip-distance apart (or slightly wider than hip-distance apart). Hold between 1 and 4 kg dumb-bells in your hands (depending on your strength levels). Arms down by your side and palms facing forward.

How to: Inhale slowly and lower yourself towards the ground by bending your knees. At the same time, bend the elbows and bring the dumb-bells up by performing a bicep curl motion. Exhale slowly, straighten the knees and bring the arms back to starting position. Do 15–20 repetitions.

What are you working: Glutes, biceps, shoulder stabilizers, core, quadriceps and calves.

Keep in mind: Remember to squat by pushing your bum back and not by bringing the knees forward. You can lean forward a bit, but try not to curl the pelvis or round the back.

5. Bird dog

Starting position: For this exercise, you have to be on all fours. Use a mat. Start kneeling with your knees under your hips and your hands under your shoulders. Keep your core engaged and your back in a neutral position.

How to: Inhale to prepare, keep the core engaged, maintain the natural curve of the spine. Exhale. Lift one leg off the mat, straightening the knee and lifting the leg as high as possible without extending the spine. Inhale. Bring the leg back under the hip, but don't put the knee down. Repeat this 15–20 times on the same side. On the last repetition, keep your leg out and pulse the leg up and down 20 times. Repeat this with the other leg.

What are you working: Core, glutes, hamstrings, lower back, shoulder stabilizers and obliques to ensure stability.

Keep in mind: Do not let the back extend when you straighten the leg, keep the core engaged and back neutral. Don't just kick the leg out and bring it in, consciously engage your glutes and focus on the muscle. Also ensure your elbows are not hyperextended.

Second trimester

1. Side leg raises

Starting position: Lie on your side, ensuring the body is in a straight line from head to toe. Relax your head on the bottom arm. Ensure your core is engaged and you are not sinking into the mat. Inhale.

How to: There are three easy to moderate level variations of this exercise:
- *Straight up:* Exhale. Slowly lift the top leg, keeping your core engaged and glutes squeezed. Inhale. Lower the leg. Go slow – it's not as much about taking the leg high as it is about keeping the core engaged and the glutes squeezed. Avoid falling forward or back. Do 10–20 repetitions on each leg.

- *Circle:* Lift the top leg and make a circle in the air – take your leg forward only as much as you can take it back. Remember to breathe throughout and try not to rock the body forward and back. Do 10 repetitions each clockwise and anti-clockwise. Do the full set on the other side.
- *Lift both legs together:* Keep your feet together. Exhale. Lift both legs up. Inhale. Lower them back to the mat. Do 10–20 repetitions.

What are you working: The hip extensors as well as hip flexors. The abductors, glutes and core. This exercise also works the obliques and multifidus to stabilize the torso.

Keep in mind: The body should be in a straight line throughout. So, at the start, relax your head on the bottom arm and not the palm, as this changes the alignment and causes undue tension on your wrist.

2. Bird dog and hamstring curls

Starting position: For this exercise, you have to be on all fours. Use a mat. Start by kneeling with your knees under your hips and your hands under your shoulders. Keep your core engaged and your back in a neutral position.

How to: Inhale to prepare, keep the core engaged, maintain the natural curve of the spine. Exhale. Lift one leg off the mat, straighten the knee and lift the leg as high as possible without extending the spine. Inhale. Bring the leg back, under the hip, but don't put the knee down. Repeat 15–20 times on the same side. At the end of the repetitions, on the last repetition, keep your leg out and pulse the leg up and down 20 times. After the pulses, perform the hamstring curls. Inhale to stay with your leg straight, knee at hip height, glute squeezed and core engaged. Exhale. Bend the knee and try to get your heel to your glute without letting the knee drop or your hips twist. Inhale. Extend the knee. Repeat with the other leg.

What are you working: Core, glutes, hamstrings, lower back, shoulder stabilizers and obliques to ensure stability.

Keep in mind: Do not let the back extend when you straighten the leg; keep the core engaged and back neutral. Don't just kick the leg out and bring it in. Consciously engage your glutes and focus on the muscle. Also ensure your elbows are not hyperextended. In the hamstring curl, it is also important to focus on keeping the leg high, without extending the back.

3. Hip flexor and quad stretch

Starting position: Start by kneeling on one knee and place the other foot forward. Be close to something you can hold on to or put your hands on the front leg or knee for support. You can kneel on a towel or thin cushion for added comfort under the knee.

How to: Inhale to stay. Exhale and slowly push the hips forward as much as you can to feel a stretch on the hip flexors and quads. Breathe deeply and hold the stretch for 15–30 seconds. Repeat on the other side.

What are you working: This stretches the hip flexors and quads and thus helps take some pressure off the lower back and spine too.

Keep in mind: Only stretch as far as you are comfortable. Don't overstretch. Also, stay close to something so you can take support as and when needed.

4. Single-arm row plus triceps kick-back

Starting position: You will need a dumb-bell for this exercise, or you could use a water bottle or anything with some amount of weight that you can hold easily in your hand. Stand in a lunge-like position, with the front knee bent and over the ankle and the back knee straight. Lean slightly forward. Hold the dumb-bell in one hand. You can keep the free hand on your thigh for support or stay close to something in case you need additional balance. Keep your core engaged throughout.

How to: Inhale to stay and keep the dumb-bell hand straight by your side, elbow extended. Exhale. Bend your elbow and drive it to the ceiling while bringing your shoulder blade back, hence lifting the dumb-bell up. After this movement, keep the elbow high and extend it back and upwards, focusing on the triceps. Inhale, bend the elbow while keeping it high, then straighten it downwards, bringing it back to the starting position. Exhale. Repeat. Do 15–20 repetitions on each side. Focus on your breath and move slowly.

What are you working: Back, shoulders, triceps, biceps, hips and core stability.

Keep in mind: Avoid rounding or arching your spine; focus on keeping your spine neutral. Don't rush the movement. There are four distinct movements, so focus on all four. Don't overextend the elbow at any point and also try not to sink or rotate at the hip or torso.

5. Triceps push-ups

Starting position: Start in a high plank position, with your hands directly under your shoulders. Keep your legs straight and hips level. Engage your core.

How to: Inhale and lower yourself towards the ground by bending your elbows and bringing your arms close to your sides, so that your elbows are pointed back. Go as low as you can, ideally until your arms, shoulders and elbows make a 90-degree angle. Exhale. Push into your hands to lift your body back up. Do 15–20 repetitions.

Modification: The same movement can be done with your knees resting down on the ground or even against a wall, depending on your fitness level.

What are you working: Triceps, chest, shoulders and core.

Keep in mind: Don't let your hips drop or stay up. Your body should lower itself and lift up in one straight line; nothing should be left behind. If the knees are down, a very common mistake is to leave the bum up while doing this exercise; try and avoid that. The body must go down and come up as a whole. Don't let your elbows hyperextend in the plank position.

Third trimester

1. Sumo squat plus pulse

Starting position: Stand with your feet about shoulder-distance apart. The feet should be turned out (laterally rotated from the hip) and back straight. Keep your core engaged and arms relaxed by your side or in front of your chest together.

How to: Inhale to lower yourself towards the ground, keep your back straight and ensure your knees are right over your ankles. Exhale. Engage your glutes, press into your feet and slowly come back up to the starting position. Do 15–20 repetitions. On the last repetition, stay down and pulse (small movements) up and down 20 times.

What are you working: The glutes, hamstrings, quadriceps and inner thighs.

Keep in mind: Don't let your knees fall inwards while doing the sumo squat. Keep them over the ankle and turned outwards. Try not to lean forward; your back should be neutral and straight.

2. Side lunges

Starting position: Start standing, with your feet more than shoulder-distance apart. Keep your feet parallel or slightly turned out. Keep your arms relaxed, core engaged and back in neutral.

How to: Inhale. Sit towards one leg, pushing the hips back a bit and bending the knee. The opposite knee stays straight and the inner thigh gets a mild stretch. Exhale. Squeeze your glutes and come back to standing position.

What are you working: Adductor, abductor, glutes, quadriceps, core and back.

Keep in mind: Don't push the knee forward, push the hip back. Try not to curl the spine and remember to keep your core engaged throughout. Don't let your feet lift off the floor. Equally distribute weight between both feet.

3. Donkey kicks

Starting position: For this exercise, you have to be on all fours. Use a mat. Start by kneeling with your knees under your hips and hands under your shoulders. Keep your core engaged and back in a neutral position.

How to: Inhale to prepare. Exhale and keep the knee bent and lift one leg up – think of pushing the ceiling or tearing through the sky with your heel. Inhale. Bring the leg back down, without putting the knee on the ground.

What are you working: Glutes, core, back, shoulder stabilizers and hamstrings.

Keep in mind: Don't let the back extend. Keep your core engaged throughout and don't overextend the elbows.

4. Standing side leg raises

Starting position: Start with your hands out in front of you or resting on your hips. Stand upright with your toes facing forward.

How to: There are two easy- to moderate-level variations of this exercise:

- Straight up: Exhale. Slowly lift one leg up and out, keeping your core engaged and glutes squeezed. Inhale. Lower the leg. Go slow – it's not as much about taking the leg higher as it is about keeping the core engaged and the glutes squeezed. Avoid leaning forward or back. Do 10–20 repetitions on each leg and then pulse for 20 repetitions.
- Circle: Lift the top leg and make a circle in the air – take your leg forward only as much as you can take it back. Remember to breathe throughout and try not to rock the body forward and back. Do 10 repetitions each clockwise and anticlockwise. Do the full set on the other side.

What are you working: Hip extensors as well as hip flexors and abductors, glutes and core. This exercise also works the obliques and multifidus to stabilize the torso.

Keep in mind: Don't rock the body. Keep your glutes squeezed throughout and try not to kick the leg up, but instead actually squeeze the glutes and slowly lift the leg as high as possible. It is similar to the side leg raises, just standing. If you want to up the intensity, you can add ankle weights or a resistance band around the ankle. Also, stay close to a wall or a chair for support, as this also challenges your balance.

5. Forward raise

Starting position: For this exercise you will need two dumb-bells or two water bottles of equal weight. Stand with your feet about shoulder-width apart, back straight and arms holding the weights. The palms face back towards the thighs, and the hands are in front of the thighs. Keep the core engaged.

How to: Exhale. Lift the weights upwards, arms out in front and palms facing down, up to shoulder level. Keep the elbows a bit soft (slightly bent) to reduce stress on the joints. Inhale slowly, with control, lower the dumb-bells back to the starting position. Do 10–20 repetitions.

What are you working: Shoulders, chest and core stability.

Keep in mind: Ensure you are not swinging the weights up. Keep the core engaged and lift your arms up without rocking the pelvis or throwing the dumb-bells up.

10

SELF-CARE

My beauty routine

Want a confession? I didn't think I looked especially attractive during many months of my pregnancy with Jeh, especially in the first trimester. And remember my first trimester the second time around was so much worse. The baby-making process sucked me of all my energy. I had puffy under-eye dark circles. I also got dry patches on my face. During Taimur's time, I was younger, more outgoing; I wanted to dress up, to wear make-up, to look pretty and to party.

By the last trimester though with both my pregnancies, I didn't look or feel especially sexy. My stomach was popping out, my thighs had ballooned and my legs got really huge. The added weight on my legs led to spider veins, and my ankles looked like two balls. Luckily I never got any stretch marks on my tummy. But that is a genetic predisposition. My mother and sister never got stretch marks, nor did my nani before us. If I was meant to get stretch marks, I would have! No fancy stretch mark cream in the world would have stopped it from happening.

My attitude was not to get too stressed about the changes in my body. I knew I could do nothing about it, and didn't get too hung up over it. In fact you probably think I spend hours every week on my skin, hair and beauty. But I really don't! I have just a few simple beauty rituals. Nor am I into those fancy beauty products with all their AHAs and retinols. The 'Made in Paris' stuff just never worked for me.

I use very general off-the-shelf kind of stuff – local home-grown products and a simple moisturizer on my skin. You won't ever bump into me in the Harrods beauty hall, picking up the latest night serums or beauty masks. I really feel many of these internationally manufactured products do not work for Indian skin. Even Saif has more toiletries than I do.

Instead, my dermatologist is my kitchen and my cook! I truly believe in home remedies. There is nothing like a simple papaya and dahi mask. I use freshly mashed papaya with its seeds on my face. It is so cooling, so soothing. I also use cucumber slices to relax my eyes. I use up whatever I find in my fridge to put on my face and skin. I also put chane ka atta and multani mitti on my skin. Are these things an essential part of my so-called beauty regimen? No! I did these things as and when I pleased, probably once in 15 days. It didn't consume me. I don't think a beauty routine would have changed the way I looked.

For my body, I swear by a concoction of almond oil and dahi. During both my pregnancies, I mixed it up (about two spoons each) and used it on my thighs, tummy and breasts. I use this on Taimur too. Just simple homemade dahi and almond oil. Nothing fancy. I have a local guy who makes me fresh cold-pressed almond oil. There are so many oil pressers available across our towns and cities who can do this for you. It really softened my skin.

When my feet would swell up, I'd just soak them in a tub of warm salted water. Simple and effective. My other home beauty ritual is oiling my hair. I love my warm oil champis. I am diligent about it and do it once in 10 to 15 days. I use a concoction of coconut oil, almond oil and olive oil all heated up together nicely with a spoon of methi seeds. Methi seeds are super for hair. My mother always used this oil on herself, and I do the same.

During Jeh's time, I broke out in spots and acne; something that's never happened to me before. Don't laugh when you read this, but I used good old toothpaste on my acne spots. The old-school Indian teenager trick. I was patient with myself. And you have to be too. I knew this was happening because of the hormonal flux in my body. My short stress-free holiday in the cool mountain air of Dharamshala helped too. My skin just cleared up and improved on its own in three to four months. Later, in my last trimester during Jeh's time, my skin looked pretty tired. You might even spot it in the cover of this book, which I shot just two weeks before I gave birth. There was nothing I could do about it though. It was a combination of exhaustion and sleepless nights.

My pregnancy style

During both my pregnancies, I got big. But that didn't stop me from liking the way I carried myself. Like most women, I was very excited to buy new maternity clothes during my first pregnancy. I picked up Gucci, Saint Laurent and other expensive maternity wear. I partied a lot, wore glamorous dresses and I rocked my heels. I remember one party I went to with Saif, where I wore this gorgeous one-shoulder olive-coloured gown with a high slit and gold gladiator heels. It was probably one of the most circulated photographs of my pregnancy! I worked a lot with stylist Anaita Shroff Adajania during Taimur's time.

I did try and hold off as far as I could from picking up 'maternity' wear. It was during my fifth month that I gave in for the first time and picked up maternity pants! Amongst the first things I did during both my pregnancies was swap out my lingerie for comfortable, cotton (and, yes, larger sized) Marks & Spencer bras and underwear. That's the way I roll, ladies! In my granny undies.

My second pregnancy was far less glamorous. Jeh's time was spent mid-pandemic and pretty locked down. I had stylist Tanya Ghavri assisting me through it. I didn't touch my jeans for months on end. They were all chucked to the back of my wardrobe. I went with lots of kaftans, loose dresses, comfortable Indian wear, slip-on shoes and Kolhapuri chappals. I wore lovely new home-grown designer labels from lots of upcoming designers. I practically lived in my cotton kaftans.

I had one great shoot through this pregnancy. It was for the Puma campaign in my last trimester. I wore tight clothes and didn't mind 'looking fat'. I couldn't shy away from that. I think the crew was more hesitant than I was. I told them I am not a supermodel. Hey, if you have a fit and active pregnancy and you plan to work out, walk and do yoga, you need those well-fitted and comfortable workout clothes, right? So go ahead! I explicitly asked the company not to 'touch up' these photographs. And the pictures came out just great. If my pregnancy weight journey can give even a few women some body goals, I'll be thrilled.

Kareena is a good UK 8 on a normal day. She fits sample sizes. But I remember the first time I saw her, post Taimur. As her stylist, when I saw her post-baby weight gain, I got pretty nervous. But in six months, she looked smoking! She had walked the ramp for Anita Dongre very shortly after she had Taimur. It was an anarkali kurta. At that time, it was tricky designing things for her. Contrary to how she looked on the ramp, she didn't feel confident that day. When she looked back on it, she swore the look didn't work for her. But she is a thorough professional. No matter what, she doesn't back out of her commitments. I never even realized she was ranked amongst the top few Indian celebrities for endorsements last year while she was pregnant with Jeh, at the height of the pandemic!

She may not be proud of every look of hers that was photographed during her pregnancies, but she is the only Indian celebrity in my books who really owned her pregnancies. What I admire about her is that she has always embraced the different phases of her life. Whether it was during her pregnancy, post baby or her time at the gym. She has never gone into a shell or hidden herself away. I have seen her through her skinniest to her biggest and back.

Like any girl, she was excited about her first pregnancy. Kareena was all around town during her pregnancy with Taimur, in plunge necks, in Gucci, in Saint Laurent. I'll never forget her in that fitted trench dress and strappy black five-inch heels styled by Anaita Shroff Adajania. During her second pregnancy, she had very few occasions to dress for. Given the lockdown situation, I think she just found it silly to dress up! Posting photographs of herself in her various kaftans became her statement. Jeh's pregnancy was all about easy styles, loose fits, lots of prints, shift dresses, kaftans and Indian clothes. I saw her in a lot of Anita Dongre, Shruti Sancheti and Masaba. I particularly loved the Rajdeep Ranawat Indian outfit she wore for Saif's birthday. — TANYA GHAVRI, celebrity stylist

Gosh, she has really carried her pregnancies beautifully! The few of us who are really close to her put on weight with her during both her pregnancies. It was a pseudo-pregnancy for me too. We would cook for her, cater to her whims, eat together, and spend hours chilling. The only time I actually saw her look tired was during the eighth and ninth months of her pregnancy with Jeh. We have had such laughs! During both her pregnancies, I would continually have to remind her 'to sit like a lady'. And she would just roll her eyes and say, 'I can't hack my thunder thighs.'

She was never guilty about enjoying her pizzas and burping. She was a trooper. Kareena was always on her feet, getting out there and doing her thing. She always looked amazing in my books. I recall that one-shoulder olive gown with a high slit and gold gladiator heels she wore during Taimur's pregnancy. She had such flair. I even remember asking her why she was wearing heels! But she was strutting with the utmost confidence. And during Jeh's time: well, the number of kaftans she wore! Once he was born, I told her to make a bonfire and burn them! — MALAIKA ARORA

What to wear when you're expecting

You might be a mom who wants a bit of fun shopping for herself and who is happy picking up a few new outfits. Enjoy this moment and enjoy your clothes! But some of you might feel worried about spending more money. The good news is you really don't need to do a great deal of shopping for maternity clothes – if you don't want to, that is. Some moms, depending on weight gain and body shape, end up doing no shopping at all.

If you've been fairly fit and active before your pregnancy, your body shape isn't going to alter that quickly. In fact, most moms don't really need to go up a size till their fifth month. Typically, it is at about 18–20 weeks of your pregnancy, when your uterus moves upwards and lines up with your navel, that you may suddenly feel like your tops aren't covering your belly and those pants aren't zipping up. You can, however, stretch out your existing stock of clothes and underwear till the time you can.

In this section we'll look at the essential new clothes you'll need during pregnancy, i.e., the few comfortable and sensible items that will get you through the next one-odd year post pregnancy too – while you nurse, juggle your baby, get back to work, and as your size continues to change. One piece of advice: whatever you buy, try and get high quality products that don't wear out fast and that support you. For instance, badly made maternity pants with belly bands can have an annoying habit of becoming loose.

Most of us continue to remain conservative about our growing belly and don't necessarily want it to peek out. That's absolutely fine. Your pregnancy wardrobe should essentially make you feel comfortable at all times. So, check the bump, the cleavage and the panty line to make sure you feel right about them. But don't get hassled about concealing your bump with loose clothes or trying to minimize it. No one is going to worry about your stomach sticking out, and neither should you.

First off, Marie Kondo your own wardrobe

Check your pre-existing kurtas, comfortable salwars and palazzos, tunics, loose joggers/sweatpants, leggings, oversized shirts, button-down tops, empire-waist tops and dresses, maxi skirts, long dresses and elastic-waist pants. A simple kaftan and loose shirt will take you through many nights and days of your pregnancy and the hazy and tiring postnatal period too. You could also consider taking your trusted salwars to the tailors and having them elasticated. Many moms find that the usual drawstring salwars slip off their bump.

A little hack that many moms use to wear their pre-pregnancy jeans and trousers for as long as they can is this: grab a rubber band (those big stationery store rubber bands) and loop it around your button, through the eye and hook it back. You'll be able to get a secure fit even though those buttons don't close.

This is also a great time to rifle through the closets of your husband, dad, brother or friend and borrow a couple of men's T-shirts or shirts – the shirt might work well with a pair of maternity jeans and the T-shirt for your daily fitness routine. There is absolutely nothing wrong with borrowing things from your mom, mom-in-law, sister or friends.

What should your essential shopping list look like?

If you are going with the streamlined approach and buying only what's strictly necessary, think about what gaps you have in outfits for your daily life – for example, professional-looking clothes for work, exercise clothes which give you proper support and so on.

A few sets of comfortable maternity jeans, leggings or pants will help. Post five months, most moms find that their existing pants either don't fit or slip off. Maternity pants are pants that stay up over your bump and give you extra support on your belly. Some even support the back. They are also designed to be extra comfortable. Now, will these pants continue to work for you a few months after delivery too, when your body is still puffy and possibly scarred (and healing)? It depends. While some moms do find their maternity pants useful for a few months post delivery, there are still many others who find no use at all for pants with belly bands the moment the baby is out and their stomach starts receding, and more so if they have a Caesarean dressing in the way. Simple elasticized- and drawstring-waist pants may work best at this stage. So do keep that in mind during your maternity shopping.

Your shirt doesn't button and your T-shirt keeps riding up? These are genuine problems! And it happens to everyone as their belly gets bigger. Three to four long T-shirts or singlets in a stretch fabric can be very handy and can be pulled down over your growing belly. There are stretchy maternity T-shirts and tops that are also slightly long which will do the same work, though you can buy these styles from non-maternity-wear lines as well. The only rule is that they should be soft and stretchy, and slightly long. Tops which have a ruched line at the sides (these ruches allow your clothes to expand with ease) will prove useful for a while.

Maternity bras are the single most important purchase you will need to make. More on this below.

Finally, you might have an office job that requires slightly more formal wear on occasion and you might need to buy new clothes for that. For these, you can consider simply going up a size or even two at your regular brands, rather than 'maternity' clothes, so that it blends with your normal sense of style. The great thing about that is you'll continue feeling like 'yourself', and when your body retreats back somewhat post delivery, you always have your good old local tailor to take in a couple of inches. Follow this advice for any other items you might need to buy too.

It would actually be ideal to choose maternity clothes that are also nursing-friendly later in your pregnancy. A sensible button-down top, an empire-waist shirt, a loose kurta or a wraparound dress or two will accommodate your growing belly and be a handy outfit to nurse your baby in later. And three solid pairs of leggings (either maternity – in case you're also exercising – or regular elastic-waist) that you can keep rotating will also take you a long way.

Wedding in the family?

What happens if you need to shop for a special occasion – like a wedding or an event? You will be understandably stressed. Nothing in your wardrobe may fit. But you can always borrow an outfit or two! Apart from that, opt for an anarkali style kurta or get a simple new blouse made for that old lovely saree or lehenga – and allow your dupatta to do the trick. If you need that one special dress or gown, by all means pick it up. However, when you're shopping for something new (and expensive) for an occasion, do try and look for an item that you will like whether you're pregnant or not. It can be altered for you later.

Exercising much?

If you happen to be working out regularly, then trackpants or tights with belly bands for extra support would be a value-add. And always pick a well-supported bra when you're exercising – keep minimum two of these if you are working out regularly. A few new maternity bras are definitely a solid buy (see section 'Shopping for the right bra'). Pick up or borrow a couple of T-shirts in bigger sizes for your walks, yoga or workouts. If you are a swimmer, a maternity swimsuit is definitely a must-have. A good maternity swimsuit is one that is: (a) lined, (b) has a covered bottom (to adjust to your growing hips), (c) has adjustable straps (to accommodate your growing size), (d) has padded cups that are removable (so you can choose how much support you need), (e) has extra pleats on the abdomen or a ruched elasticized line on the sides that can expand as you grow (for one-piece swimsuits and tankinis).

Choosing a fabric? Pick what feels light

You will really just want to wear things that feel good against your skin. Whenever and wherever you can, opt for cottons, linens and light blends. Many moms say they really just want clothes that feel soft or light against their skin. We live in a country that is largely tropical and fairly humid (which is an understatement). Lycra/Spandex isn't going to keep you very cheerful. And let's not forget how hot you feel anyway during your pregnancy! Being cool and staying cool is the only way to do this. If you're sweating a lot in your clothes, you're at risk of fungal infections (see box 'Will tight pants hurt my baby?').

While it may sound like a stretch, when you pick the simpler and more homely options, you are also precluding the need for dry cleaning too many of your clothes. Dry cleaning requires chemical solvents that can ultimately affect your already sensitive skin. As far as possible, choose to launder your clothes in water.

WILL TIGHT PANTS HURT MY BABY?

Can tight pants, fitted waistbands, belts or body-hugging clothes harm your baby? No. Can they actually cut off circulation in your body? Your clothes will have to be seriously corset-tight for that to happen! But over-tight clothes can constrict your abdomen just enough for digestion to get difficult and exacerbate those feelings of nausea, breathlessness and heartburn. So figure out your comfort level first. If you can rage in those skinny jeans, why not? But keep the season in mind. We live in a humid country and tend to sweat more. Furthermore, in India, there is a strong chance of getting ringworm. When you dress tight and your body is also bigger, you'll anyway be sweating more. The moisture attracts fungus. And ringworm infections can happen. It's tough to treat fungal infections as medication in pregnancy is as it is limited. And the problem isn't just that you have it; it's that it's contagious, and you can spread it to your family. Hygiene is important. Tight clothes are okay if the fabric is good and if you're in a cool/air-conditioned environment. Remember, through all this your baby will be fine. But if your groin and the folds of your skin break into an infection, it's just going to be a whole new bother.

(With inputs from Dr Deepti Ghia)

Footwear

Don't be surprised to find that your feet have gone up a size or so during pregnancy. This will fix itself post delivery, but in some cases there are moms who have permanently gotten stuck with half-size bigger feet. So, along with some new clothes, you might find you have to go shoe shopping as well. Look for a sensible pair of slip-on footwear (a half size bigger would help too) with padded lining, shock-absorbent soles and open toes. Why so specific, you wonder? Open toes give you room for swelling. Slip-ons ensure you're not trying to bend at odd angles to lift that back strap, fasten a buckle or tie a shoelace. And padding minimizes the friction that your increasing weight and changing posture puts on the balls and heels of your foot. If you're exercising or travelling during your pregnancy, you will need a good pair of sneakers. Don't compromise on those. Buy a sensible pair of sneakers about one to one and a half sizes bigger than your current size, depending on how big your feet get. As we have mentioned even for clothes, don't be shy to borrow – especially if it is fancy occasion wear. And when it comes to the big mommy question – heels – do what feels comfortable for you (see box 'Can I wear heels?').

Can I wear heels?

You will hear most people advising you to ditch those heels for comfortable flat shoes. There are many reasons for skipping heels, all stemming from practicality. Let's take a look.

(1) Your centre of gravity shifts as your stomach grows, which could make you feel imbalanced; (2) you may already be walking a little unsteadily (pregnancy waddle), with your legs wider apart; (3) because of your increasing body weight and hormones affecting your joints and ligaments, your knees or ankles may be a little weakened; (4) quite simply, you can just trip and fall; (5) your calf muscles can contract and lead to leg cramps, which you don't want to have to deal with; (6) if your heels invariably make you slouch a little, it could lead to back pain – which, again, you don't want to deal with; (7) the excess fluid retention in your body may make your feet and ankles swell; (8) you may have lumbar lordosis. What's that? As you know, your spine curves naturally. But, during pregnancy, the lower back curvature of your spine can get pronounced, i.e., naturally exaggerated; especially post the fifth month. It can throw you off balance.

But the point is – it is really up to you. If you have always been a heel wearer, you could most likely pull off heels comfortably, more so in your first and second trimesters. So go for it. While pencil heels and stilettos are likelier to affect your posture adversely, a pair of platform heels will distribute your body pressure evenly across your foot. Long hours of standing and varicose veins can also be exacerbated by heels. Also, the increased weight of your body puts more pressure (friction) on certain parts of your foot – especially with heels – like the balls of your feet. You could then develop corns. Heels are not going to harm your baby. It is more about your comfort. If you're not a habitual heel wearer, now may not be the right time to start.

(With inputs from Dr Deepti Ghia)

Shopping for the right bras

When you're chalking up your shopping list, what you will quite likely need is new underwear in larger sizes. By all means go for it. There are no guidelines here. Please note, however, that now is not the time to wear tight bodyshaping underwear – so do avoid it.

But when it comes to your bra – that's a game changer. It is the most important purchase of your pregnancy wardrobe. Your bra size is going to alter. That is for sure. In the very beginning, before buying a new bra, pick up a few bra extenders (easily available online and at local lingerie stores). A bra extender will work for you till the time your cup size changes significantly, but don't expect your old bras to give you the same support at this time. You will need new bras. Most moms find that they need a new bra in their altered size post 18 to 20 weeks of pregnancy.

Maternity bras: The best advice is to pick up good quality bras. Spend those few extra bucks on them, but buy bras that will last you through your pregnancy. That will truly be value for money. If you plan your sizing a little sensibly, you may not need to shop for bras more than twice during your pregnancy.

In the early stages, when you need to swap to a maternity bra for the first time (approximately midway into your second trimester), look for a soft and stretchy cup area (i.e., a bra that is in stretchy 'non-cup' sizes). It's ideal when you don't want to get limited by cup sizes. Your cup size will change more in the first few months of your pregnancy. Later on in the pregnancy, it is more about your expanding ribcage. Your bra band is also important (see 'The key factors in buying a new bra' below for more advice). Depending on how active you are and the climate you live in, you will need two to three maternity bras, especially if you regularly sleep in them.

Nursing bras: Later in your pregnancy, during what is round two (hopefully) in the third trimester, pick good quality nursing bras. A nursing bra has an unobtrusive set of clasped openings that allow you to nurse your baby with ease. It will be totally worth the money as these bras will last you through the final stretch of your 40 weeks and then through your nursing period. You should need two to three nursing bras. Again, the number depends on the climate you live in, if you need a bra to sleep in, how active you are while nursing (i.e., are you going to walk, exercise, gym), and whether or not you also have additional hands-free pumping bras.

Some moms may find that they don't need to buy bras twice over, but just move to nursing bras directly.

The key factors in buying a new bra

Here's a checklist:
- The most sensible thing would be to get bras that will lend you full support during your day and while you work out, and yet be comfortable enough for you to sleep in. Many pregnant moms find they need to sleep with a bra on to support their heavy and tender breasts. Similarly for lactating moms.

- Your maternity and nursing bras should not be underwired (as that is not comfortable for most moms through the third trimester and while breastfeeding). Look for bras where the inner cup lining is soft – your breasts may be tender during pregnancy and your nipples may be chafed while you acclimatize them to breastfeeding. Your bra shouldn't aggravate your skin.
- Both types of bras should have a soft, cushioned, adjustable and pliant band to accommodate your growing ribcage during pregnancy and, later on, your receding chest size. It is best if the band is thick and the back closure has a good secure grip (the two-hook grips won't do here). These parameters will also ensure that your bra doesn't keep riding up your back. That can be super uncomfortable.
- A good maternity and nursing bra is a 'full-support one' – mainly because your breasts will be bigger, more sensitive, tender and also heavy at the time you're lactating.

Caring for yourself

Your pregnancy is a delicate time, and you'd rather err on the side of caution through your nine months. There are so many questions every pregnant mom has, so many little things that you need to consider with care while you're carrying your little one. While we have discussed a variety of issues related to skin, hair and massages through Part 1: Your 40 Weeks, this is where we take a deep dive into all the possible salient points of pregnancy self-care.

Note: Do bear in mind at this point that your pregnancy is the time to be utterly careful. It is safe to continue using most of your simple OTC beauty products. However, check your labels for harmful ingredients (see box 'Read your labels: Retinols and other skincare ingredients to avoid'). When it comes to specialized ointments, medicines or treatments, not every drug or beauty product is studied from the pregnancy angle. There are categories of pregnancy-safe medicines and ointments. It is best to use only those. Your dermatologist, your GP, your ob-gyn or any specialist you consult will always write a prescription for you with utmost care. If you have any doubts, feel free to question your doctor.

Part 1: Face

Your hormones are in flux during pregnancy. These hormones translate to different things for different women. Let's take a look at the problems and what we can do. While many moms will experience the legendary 'pregnancy glow', for many other women, their skin actually worsens. And the biggest challenge is that you cannot medicate freely. You may find areas of hyper-pigmentation on your face too. Not every woman will go through these issues, however. And, for those who do, there is little you can do about it while you're pregnant!

Pregnancy acne
You don't have to have acne-prone skin to get pregnancy acne and breakouts. It just depends on how your body takes to pregnancy and your churn of hormones. Acne is more common in the first and second trimesters. It often resolves itself on its own.

Why does it happen? It's pretty straightforward. An increase in testosterone and androgens in your body can enhance your skin's sebum secreting powers which results in oilier skin. (So, does acne mean you're having a boy then? Maybe! But you really never know!) Oil can clog your pores and lead to breakouts, bacteria and inflammation. Pregnancy acne clears up on its own either during the course of your pregnancy or post delivery, when your hormones commence their retreat to normal.

What can I do? Apart from keeping up with your nutrition and hydration, skip sugary and salty foods and go very easy on caffeine. Remember not to overwash, overscrub or overdry your face. Be gentle when you dab your skin dry or while you use any moisturizer, toner or oil on your face. Never exfoliate your face with scrubs. In fact, as a rule of thumb, don't touch your face too much. Your hands can transfer bacteria to your already sensitive facial skin. A spot of stress, exhaustion and lack of sleep can also affect your skin. If you have an oily scalp, wash your hair frequently. Be wary about the make-up you put on your face – check your labels for non-comedogenic or hypoallergenic qualities. And, finally, keep changing your linen regularly – especially face napkins, bath towels and pillow covers.

Is there any medication? Very severe acne may need oral antibiotics which are pregnancy safe, like erythromycin and azitgromycin. Mild to moderate acne can be treated with topical (i.e., applied) antibiotics, azelaic acid and glycolic acid if it doesn't resolve on its own. But wait it out, if you can. Vitamin A and salicylic acid (usually used for face treatments) are both avoidable during pregnancy. And for those scars and that post-acne pigmentation, wait till you deliver your baby and then address them with a dermatologist.

Melasma

A common hyperpigmentation that happens during pregnancy is melasma (also called chloasma). In this case, brown patches appear on the forehead, cheeks, nose or chin. Again, these are harmless. This is a reaction to sun sensitivity combined with oestrogen and progesterone. A good (physical) sunscreen and azelaic acid topical formations can be used on your skin during pregnancy for melasma (see section 'Do I need to go "organic"?').

CAN I GET A FACIAL?

It is absolutely okay to pamper yourself when you're pregnant. A simple facial massage with fresh fruit, a skin polishing treatment, mask application and a clean-up is fine. But always be wary about what is being applied on you. Your skin is probably more sensitive than normal during your pregnancy – so, baby steps! Do be careful about 'application treatments' – for instance, while glycolic acid and azelaic acid are fine, salicylic acid is not 100 per cent pregnancy safe. Lasers and light therapy have no contraindications for your pregnancy or your baby either. But your dermatologist may ask you to avoid them completely. Why is that? While the laser rays per se are not a problem, it is how the laser machine generates those rays that is the grey area of doubt. It might actually be better for you to avoid laser rooms. If your skin is sensitive or you have acne, don't ruffle things up much. Wait it out or speak to a dermatologist. It is best not to go with the advice of your local salon facialist at this point.

DO I NEED TO SEE MY DENTIST?

Dental care may be far from your mind during these nine months, but don't skip this appointment. A great many pregnant women get gingivitis, periodontitis and gingival epulus. These issues crop up during the second and third trimesters when your hormones are rising significantly. Oral care is actually pretty important in your pregnancy, and you have to be mindful of your dental hygiene routine twice a day: brush, floss, clean your tongue. Pregnant women with periodontal disease can give birth to preterm/low birth weight babies. If you have had a long bout of morning sickness earlier on in your pregnancy accompanied with vomiting and acid reflux, it might have caused some erosion of the tooth enamel too.

Part 2: Hair

A head oil massage, a salon wash and blow-dry, and various hot tools for your hair are all pregnancy safe. Now, what about colouring your hair? And getting a chemical hair treatment? A lot of women choose to avoid all chemical treatments – and there are so many – on their hair through the nine months. It would be ideal to speak to your hair therapist and your doctor before you opt for chemical treatments on your hair. Or, simply look up the chemical components you're considering and understand the risks. And finally, when it comes to hair, possibly every pregnant mom has the same doubt and fear: the big post-birth hair loss!

Can I colour my hair?

Most hair colours and hair dyes have a chemical compound called phenylenediamine (PPD), which is amongst the most common causes of contact allergies, also called contact dermatitis (i.e., a rash that occurs because of exposure to irritating agents). During pregnancy, your immune function is altered/sensitized. Your body's immunity is designed to fight anything foreign, right? Whether it is a pathogen or a chemical, your body might react more to it. An ammonia-free range of hair colour is generally advised for pregnant women. But always know that you are taking a small risk. Your pregnancy hormones could react in unexpected ways.

Tips: Stick to the same brand you have always used. In fact, use the same combination of hair colour too. Don't change it. Line your hairline with petroleum jelly to form a barrier for your skin. Wear a mask over your nose and mouth to avoid inhaling the smell of hair colour. And if something goes wrong, see a skin doctor right away. Avoid colouring your hair for at least the first 12 weeks of pregnancy.

Are hair treatments pregnancy safe?

Most hair rebonding treatments have formalin (a colourless solution of formaldehyde in water), which is a carcinogenic compound. If possible, avoid this. Certain hair protein treatments that are formalin free are okay. Always look at the ingredients/chemicals you're going to use. Any treatments that relax and straighten the cystine bond (also called sulfur bond or disulfide bond) of your hair basically weaken it over time. So, post pregnancy, when those growth hormones have retreated and your hair is shedding again – you may not be happy. The bottom line is that you should avoid treatments that are unnecessary and non-critical.

Tips: Bear in mind the same cautions as listed for hair colour. Keep a mask on to avoid inhaling the chemical fumes. And see your doctor if you notice any adverse reactions.

Handling your post-delivery hair fall

One of the pregnancy after-effects that freak out many moms is dramatic hair loss. Here's what it means. You'll very likely enjoy a head full of lush hair through your pregnancy. Why? Basically, when you're not pregnant, it is perfectly normal for your body to shed 30–40 strands of hair per day. But your growth hormones during pregnancy essentially hold on to all those hairs that you shed daily in the routine course of things. Which is all well and good until you deliver your baby. And then? Well, three months post your baby, when your hormones have pretty much all retreated, those many strands that would have otherwise shed across 40 weeks of your life may now shed in a much shorter duration of time. And this is when you're losing those clumps of hair in the shower drain!

Can you help it? Not really! What you now need to focus on is letting your hair regenerate on its own post pregnancy. Here are a few tips that may benefit your hair health. As always, keep up with your good nutrition habits and stay hydrated through your pregnancy and way beyond too (see Chapter 8: Nutrition). Get your blood circulating with mild physical activity as soon as you're fit and able to. Stimulate your scalp with your fingers, with headstands, head massages or opt for professional hair treatments. Continue your iron and calcium supplements for several months post delivery. This is actually pretty important for any new mom. And, if you need help, see a doctor; you can start a (breastfeeding-safe) cyclical therapy of oral supplements like zinc, amino acids, B complex and antioxidants.

Can I thread and wax?

During your pregnancy, the hair on your eyebrows, upper lip and body might grow faster than it did before. And a question many women have is if they can continue to wax and thread. Yes, you can. Your sensitized skin may get itchy or red post a wax, but that can happen any time to anyone. Don't wax (or even thread) a previously untouched area of your body. And use the same type of waxing agent too. Stick to the tried and tested, as your skin may react adversely at any time.

Part 3: Body

There is a lot to talk about here, from oils and moisturizing, to stretch marks, hyperpigmentation, varicose veins and those pregnancy FAQs. And the biggest one of all? Do you need to change your body products and go 'organic'? Let's take a look.

Do I need to moisturize?

Yes! Keep your skin really hydrated and moist through your pregnancy. Your pregnancy hormones and quickly stretching skin are going to make you feel dry, itchy and, yes, prone to stretch marks. Moisturizing well from day one may not mean you won't get stretch marks (which is a natural process), but you can perhaps minimize the appearance/severity of stretch marks. How do you stay moisturized? Start with the most basic things: eat nutritious whole foods and keep up with your water intake and prenatal vitamins. Stick with the body oils you are used to (coconut oil is particularly good). Look for lotions with magnesium, ceramides, squalene, cholesterol esters, natural oils and body butters like shea, cocoa and mango butter (see sections 'Oils and massages' and 'What do I do about those stretch marks?')

QUICK TIP: FOR DRY AND ITCHY SKIN

Take one cup of coconut oil (regular or extra virgin), half cup aloe vera gel (optional) and 12 capsules of vitamin E (cut and squeeze out the medicine). Mix it well. Store it in a clean jar. Refrigerate. Apply it cold on your skin. Make it in small servings and use it fresh throughout your nine months. Always avoid using old products on your skin during pregnancy.

Oils and massages

The one thing you will need to take careful stock of is moisturizing your body during your pregnancy and keeping up with it post delivery too. Oils can be invaluable in keeping your body supple and healthy, and some oils can help tackle moisture loss. If you are getting pregnancy and postpartum massages, you will need oils as well. Dhanwantharam Thailam is a classic Ayurvedic oil for expectant and new mothers.

You should be able to use any carrier oil – these are vegetable oils from seeds and nuts that are the base oil in which essential oils are diluted to create blended massage oils. The most common carrier oils are almond, jojoba, sesame, coconut, castor, apricot, moringa and grapeseed. You should ideally buy these cold pressed.

While most of you can use any of the popular carrier oils on your body, you have to be careful about using essential oils. Essential oils are distilled from the aromatic leaves, bark and roots of plants. These are the oils that are used in very small proportions along with carrier oils to fragrance them, like lavender. Most essential oils aren't recommended during pregnancy.

Also be careful when it comes to using oils on your face. Additionally, don't go with everything that is advertised or promoted as 'good for your skin'. Olive oil, for instance, has a keratolytic action on your skin (i.e., it affects the keratin component of your skin) and forms a thick layer that doesn't absorb that easily, thereby causing problems like acne, contact dermatitis or eczema. Olive oil is great for your hair, especially if you have dandruff. Even mustard oil (sarson ka tel) has contact allergens and is avoidable for body massages. Speak to a doctor or ask a dermatologist to guide you.

There is also a handy tip on massaging right. Across trimesters one, two and three, we have talked about massages, including gentle back rubs or foot rubs done at home by a partner or a family member. The first thing to bear in mind for your massages is to use oils that are tried and tested by you. (A bottle of good moisturizer will also do for a massage.) And another key point to remember during any massage (prenatal or postnatal) – and this is especially if you have a semi-skilled maalishwali coming home for you – is that it should always be unidirectional, i.e., in the direction where the hair is growing. Otherwise it causes occlusion of the hair follicles, which can result in inflammation. Don't let anyone rub your skin up and down.

Making the most of oils during your pregnancy

With Anita Lal, creative director of Paro by Good Earth

It is important to understand the composition of our skin and the nature and key benefits of oils before using them. Our skin consists of three main layers:

- Epidermis – the outermost layer of the skin, which acts as a waterproof, protective barrier
- Dermis – middle layer of the skin where collagen and elastin are found
- Hypodermis – the deepest layer of the skin, composed of fat and connective tissue

In pregnancy, especially during the last trimester, stretch marks may form in the dermis, or middle layer, because the connective tissue is stretched beyond the limits of its elasticity. This causes the dermis to tear, allowing deeper layers of skin to show through. Collagen plays a role in keeping your skin strong and elastic and it may also be important for minimizing stretch marks. Vitamin C is an important nutrient for the development of collagen. So apart from including Vitamin C in your diet and hydrating the body with six to eight glasses of water daily, you can apply cold-pressed seed oils that are rich in vitamins and essential fatty acids which have Omegas 3-6-9.

You could select and make a blend of Omega 9-rich cold-pressed oils (from seeds) like moringa, apricot and almond in combination with Omega 6-rich oils like rosehip, sea buckthorn, sunflower, safflower, evening primrose and borage, and also Omega 3-rich oils like flaxseed and walnut seed. Most oils contain the three main Omegas in varying proportions.

Below are two simple formulations that you can make yourself and use through your pregnancy to keep your skin supple and healthy. Follow these two recipes to make a 100 ml blend of cold-pressed seed oils.

Recipe 1

35 ml sweet almond oil (for moisturizing and easy absorption)

35 ml apricot kernel oil (nutrient rich)

20 ml rosehip seed oil (boosts collagen)

5 ml flaxseed oil (calms inflammation)

3 ml borage seed oil (for healing)

2 ml wheatgerm oil (rich in vitamin E)

Recipe 2

50 ml moringa oil (nutrient rich)

30 ml safflower oil (soothes dry skin)

10 ml walnut oil (vitamin rich)

5 ml sea buckthorn oil (for cell regeneration)

5 ml evening primrose oil (to counter dryness)

In addition, you can include some safe essential oils that can add a hint of fragrance and give your skin some benefits as well.

Lavender and vetiver are calming oils that benefit the nervous system, and geranium and petitgrain are also considered safe oils. A word of caution here would be to use essential oils in very low quantities, i.e., no more than 0.5 per cent of the total oil blend.

What about those stretch marks?

Will I get them? The dreaded question! If you are genetically predisposed to stretch marks (check if your mother or grandmother have them), you will quite likely get them too. The only difference is, when. Stretch marks depend on the inherent elasticity of your skin. If they have to appear, they will. And they will most likely be across your stomach, thighs, breasts or buttocks.

What should I do? Try products which contain ceramides, squalene or cholesterol esters. These compounds are proven to actually get absorbed into your skin structure and become part of it, which helps in improving skin quality and moisturizing from within. The best thing to do from early in your pregnancy is moisturize and soothe your dry and itchy skin with a good lotion or a good quality oil (see section 'Oils and massages'). Try aloe vera/shea butter- and magnesium-based moisturizing products. Gently massage them into your skin post a bath. Avoid retinoid-based stretch mark removal creams completely (see box 'Read your labels: Retinols and other skincare ingredients to avoid').

Will they go later? If these marks really bother you post delivery, you can consult a dermatologist and explore the options of derma pen, microneedling or skin-tightening machines. Just remember that while your stretch marks may never fully disappear, they may get camouflaged. If you're super particular, don't wait for the fresh purple/red lines to turn into those dull silvery white marks; it is too late then to seek any intervention.

WORRIED ABOUT THAT BIG DARK LINE ON YOUR TUMMY?

The linea nigra shows up on a lot of pregnant women. It's nothing to worry about. It is a distinctly dark, one-cm line of hyperpigmentation going vertically up the centre of your abdomen. Why exactly it happens is unknown. It could be the pregnancy hormones that cause the skin cells to darken while high oestrogen affects the melanocyte-stimulating hormone that is made in the placenta. The linea nigra fades away post pregnancy. It is nothing more than an aesthetic inconvenience until the time it disappears on its own.

Skin darkening and skin tags

Acanthosis (hyperpigmentation on the body) and acrochordons (hangings of skin) crop up pretty commonly in pregnant Indian women. Understand what they are and what you can do.

Acanthosis: It is very common for pregnant women to develop acanthosis. Here, velvety dark or black patches begin to form at the back of your neck, in your underarms and between your thighs. These are the 'common' areas. It happens because of your hormones, weight gain, insulin resistance and metabolic change. It is harmless. Leave it alone and address it post pregnancy with lifestyle changes (exercise), insulin medication (like metformin to improve metabolism and sugar utilization), topical applications and oral medications. Post delivery, you can go aggressive with your treatment. Chances are it will lighten but will not fade away completely. It is simply an internal reaction of your skin.

Acrochordons: Skin tags are common too. These are known as acrochordons and are hangings or folds of skin that form in the underarm area, neck area or under the breasts (and occasionally in the groin area), mainly because of hormonal changes and weight gain. These tags commonly occur during menopause too. If your parents have skin tags, you're likelier to have them too. It's a genetic predisposition. Leave it alone. You can easily get rid of it post pregnancy. Your doctor will apply a numbing cream on the area of the skin tag and then use a radio frequency device to zap it out. You can remove it during pregnancy too – especially if it occurs in an area that obstructs your birth canal. For instance, if the tag is in your groin area and it is big, you may need to remove it if you're going in for a vaginal birth. During your pregnancy, your doctor is likelier to use a physical (i.e., not electrical) method for getting rid of skin tags: clamping and crushing to excise them.

I see spider veins and varicose veins

Spider veins are the tiny red veins that form on your skin because of the increased blood flow placing pressure on your vessels. However varicose veins are different and need more elaboration.

What are they? Varicose veins are the purplish/blue (bruise-coloured) veins that show up on your legs. Your growing abdomen and weight put pressure on your legs and create a sort of bottleneck to your lower body. It is, quite simply, a huge cosmetic inconvenience.

What helps? Prop your feet up when you can and maintain movement in your feet. Don't sit cross-legged. Varicose veins take a lot longer to fade post delivery and may need surgical intervention. There is no major scientific evidence that backs up the benefits of using compression socks for varicose veins during pregnancy (these socks are commonly used for varicose veins otherwise).

Can it be treated? Varicose veins can also lead to varicose eczema, by the way, which makes your skin very itchy. You may need to apply a topical medicated (eczema) ointment under the guidance of your doctor. If these vein marks greatly bother you post delivery, you can track down a superspeciality clinic that has vascular lasers and get them treated.

Why do my breasts look weird?

Your breasts may begin to grow during your pregnancy as will the areolas (the pigmented portion around the nipples), which may get larger and much darker. It is the normal flux of hormones, fat and blood volume that are affecting the glands and tissues of your breasts. Many pregnant women also notice small bumps in the areolas. These are simply oil (sebaceous) glands that usually become prominent during a menstrual cycle or pregnancy. These bumps even have an official name: Montgomery's tubercles! You can stay relaxed about this, unless you see something overtly out of place – like inverted nipples, discharge, dimpled skin or nodes, for which you must go see your doctor. And, yes, don't ignore the benefits of a good bra during your pregnancy (see section 'Shopping for the right bra').

Ugh, my feet have swollen

It is very common for pregnant women to develop swelling in their fingers, hands, ankles or feet. This has little to do with the increasing levels of progesterone in your body and a lot to do with the extra fluid accumulation in your body (oedema, which we discussed way back in trimester two) that's acting up. Can you help it? No. Is it a problem? Well, it just makes your hands, face and feet look puffy. Such swelling disappears on its own post delivery. So what can you do about it meanwhile?

- At the end of a long tiring day, prop up your feet whenever possible. In fact, when you're lying down, see if you can get your feet up a little higher than the rest of your body (use a few extra blankets and pillows for height) and spend some time in this position.

- While your feet do need some rest and elevation, you should also be maintaining your circulation with short ten-minute walks a couple of times a day and doing gentle stretches. In fact, keep up with your daily fitness activity.

- Swelling is aggravated if you've had too much caffeine or salty food. It goes without saying, up your water intake (even though you have enough 'fluid' in your body, it's not the same thing) and cut down on sugars, salts and caffeine. Up your potassium intake with the right kinds of food (like banana, dahi, sweet potato, beetroot, etc.) because potassium aides in fluid balance. Pick anti-inflammatory foods to augment your diet.

- In the warmer months of the year, dress in loose and comfortable clothes and try and keep your body temperature cool.
- Use ice packs on your swelling wherever comfortable. Ice cubes wrapped in a napkin will also do. You can soak a towel in cold water and cover your legs with it. And another simple remedy: fill up half a bucket of warm (not hot) water, add some salt/rock salt and soak your feet in it. Try a relaxing foot massage with any simple oil or moisturizer.
- Here's a quick tip: Don't shy away from comfortable sensible footwear; if you need to go up a size, pick up a good slip-on pair that will get you through a large part of your pregnancy.

If your swelling is excessive and accompanied with proteins in the urine, dizziness, blurry vision, face swelling, high blood pressure or rapid weight gain, you should consult your ob-gyn and seek medical intervention.

Should I go 'organic'?

Now, there is a lot of stuff available out there: international and local, organic and high-tech. And it's all just fine if it works for your skin. Remember that your body is ultra sensitive during pregnancy. You never know which pre-existing skin condition (like eczema, psoriasis or rosacea) can also get aggravated because of your pregnancy hormones. It is important to understand the action of every ingredient on your body. Each compound, whether natural or lab-made, has a chemical formula of its own and could have a reaction on your body. So you will have to spend some time analysing labels.

Stick with the tried-and-tested products that you have always used on your body and hair. The same goes for your make-up products too. Many pregnant moms specifically swap to products that are paraben free, hypoallergenic, sulphate free, non-comedogenic and fragrance free during their pregnancy. You can look up 'clean make-up' and 'clean beauty' labels online and do your own R&D to figure out what might work for you.

But there is no hard-and-fast rule about that. Simple OTC beauty and hygiene products that we get in any average Indian pharmacy do not have harmful amounts of chemical components. But read your labels as certain OTC moisturizers and anti-ageing creams have retinols (see box 'Read your labels: Retinols and other skincare ingredients to avoid'). Most standard, reputed cosmaceutical brands in India have chemical compositions that are rated safe as per global averages.

When products are scientifically assessed, it means they have gone through a number of critical studies. Globally, the organic cosmaceutical industry isn't very strictly bound. And not every beauty product you find out there is tested for pregnancy safety. It is best not to run with the assumption that organic or naturopathy is automatically 'safe'. If you don't understand labels, consult an expert. At the end of the day, everything around you is a chemical compound of some sort – like 'sodium chloride' when worded as 'common salt' becomes a home remedy! There is no right or wrong answer here.

Here's a quick tip on using sunscreen. Swap to a 'physical' sunscreen (which has active mineral ingredients like titanium dioxide or zinc oxide) as opposed to a 'chemical' sunscreen. A physical sunscreen sits on top of your skin like a protective layer and deflects the UV rays. It doesn't get absorbed into your skin.

Read your labels: Retinols and other skincare ingredients to avoid

If you have been using a range of specialized products, ointments or make-up, do check the labels when you conceive. There are a few chemicals that are contraindicated during pregnancy and in the pre-pregnancy/conception stage too. All dermatologists will advise you to avoid certain chemical compounds from the time you start planning your baby.

- Retin-A, retinol, retinyl palmitate: While these usually appear in prescription-based products, there are some OTC products which contain these vitamin A derivatives. Retinoids are teratogenic. While studies have not shown any problems with topical retinoids, oral retinoids have indicated teratogenicity in the baby (i.e., causing problems in growth). Other vitamin A derivatives are tazorac and accutane, which aren't good for the baby.

- Finasteride, which is found in hair medication, should not be taken when you conceive. A natural herb preparation called saw palmetto should also be avoided. Both are male hormone antagonists. In fact, if you happen to be on a course of medication like this and get pregnant, your ob-gyn will advise an immediate ultrasound, run some tests, examine the duration of time the medication has been taken and may even recommend an abortion. Incidentally, your dermatologist or family physician will tell you in advance not to conceive for a certain number of months while you are on these compounds.

- Avoid hydroquinone, which is a skin-lightening agent used for pigmentation. High amounts of salicylic acid – present in certain OTC anti-acne products – can cause salicyclism.
- Avoid deodorants and sprays with aluminium chloride hexahydrate (an antiperspirant).
- Formaldehyde/Formalin: It's a known irritant and is carcinogenic. You'll find this component in nail polish (especially gel polish) and almost all hair smoothening treatments. It is also a great preservative, which means it is used in many beauty products (and cleaning products and building materials) across the world. To assess your labels for formaldehyde releasers, look for components like methylene glycol or methanediol, DMDM hydantoin, imidazolidinyl urea, diazolidinyl urea, quaternium 15, bronidox and SHMG (sodium hydroxymethylglycinate).

Quick tips: Postnatal care for the new mom

- Get a massage: More than being eminently therapeutic, postnatal massages for the mother help her relax and calm down. Follow the same advice from the section 'Oils and massages' in this chapter.
- Avoid very hot baths as they aggravate dryness and irritation of the skin. Lukewarm water is ideal for bathing.
- When using sanitary napkins, apply a layer of your baby's nappy rash cream (like zinc oxide-based barrier

creams) on your vaginal area and the sides – i.e., external application. It simply prevents friction of your sanitary napkin against your skin and keeps rashes at bay. Always consider sanitary napkins with cotton covers for a while in the beginning.

- There may be many postpartum traditions, beliefs and rituals that your family may ask you to follow. It really is a personal thing. But do try and understand the reason why you're following certain traditions. Many families believe that a new mom should not wash her hair for the first 40 days post birth. If you are following this custom, you might want to try a dry shampoo during this time.

(With inputs from Dr Deepti Ghia)

AFTERWORD
by Saif Ali Khan

I still remember when Kareena and I first talked about our relationship seriously. It was many years ago, a casual evening. We were drinking wine and chatting on the balcony. She said she loved being with me but was worried that her work would suffer if she married and settled down. She was nervous about it. But I saw something in her. I was really surprised that she wasn't as sure as I was of the future: that she would continue to remain a huge star. She may have been fearful of commitment and family. But I knew, even then, that nothing could hold her back.

I think of Kareena as a bit of a trailblazer. Look at the choices she has made. Take our marriage. It was brave of her to decide to marry me. She was 31. I am ten years older than her. I have been married before. I have two grown-up children. It tells you what sort of person she is. If you are brave enough to make some choices in your life, you will be able to power through the odds.

And she has done that with both her pregnancies. She worked right through them. After both the kids, she started to get back into shape quickly; she jumped into work. She made it all happen. She is a crazy multitasker. She can be in hair rollers in the middle of a shoot, slip out of heels into her slippers and take a phone break to do some serious troubleshooting at home or to check in on what Taimur has eaten. She's a soldier.

My mother became an actor at sixteen. She did some outstanding work after marriage and kids. My grandmother administered a state in Bhopal, one of the few states ruled by a succession of women. The ladies in my family have shot with guns – and called the shots in more ways than one. So when I told Kareena she could do it all, I didn't just mean it flippantly. I had grown up around powerful women and genuinely believed in her.

Of course, things are pressured for a female actor in our industry. How you look is often everything! When we first began our relationship, she was at size zero, shopping in the kids' section of stores because those were the only things that would fit her. She was doing super well for herself with work, and her appearance played a big part in it. Pregnancies take their toll on your body; it takes you a while to return to shape. Kareena was worried about these things. When we first talked about having children, she even briefly wondered if she should consider a surrogate. But she then realized that everything in life needs your 100 per cent. Once she had made up her mind, she was all in.

I have seen Kareena grow from a highly strung actor (which is good for the job) to a grounded and mature woman. And she has changed as a mother too through her two pregnancies. She has a side to her that gets nervous easily. It's good, it's a careful side. When she had Taimur, she was wary of certain things. She didn't know how to pick him up, to soothe him. I carried him more and am still very connected with him, though he is very close to his mom.

With Jeh, Kareena is very different, more maternal. She holds Jeh, calms him, distracts him – she does everything she found hard the first time. It's almost like she's become another person. I suppose the lesson is to be patient with yourself. If there is anything I have learnt as a father and a partner it is that what matters is your intention. Half the trouble is when we expect too much from ourselves or from people around us.

And it's not just Kareena who has changed. Our relationship has, too. When she got pregnant, we told ourselves we would live the same life; we'd continue to travel as we always had, to Paris, London, Gstaad. We'd take our baby and maybe a nanny to help us. But life changed when Taimur was born! I know I lost interest in superficial socializing. We stayed in a lot. It brought us even closer. For us, there is nothing like getting together with our family and closest friends, having a drink with the little one running around and playing.

What hasn't changed is the fundamentals of our relationship. It has always been – and will always be – an equal one. My mother was a film star and my father was an international sportsman. I grew up watching them divide their time for their kids, and I saw the respect they had for each other's professions. My siblings and I were all brought up on their common ground. That sets the tone for Kareena and me.

When Kareena jumped back into work six months after Taimur, I was there to step in. Later this year, when she goes back to shooting for a movie, I will have finished a couple of assignments and will happily take over Jeh. It's a question of what's important to both of you. She loves her job and she's good at it. It permeates her life. It makes her a happy and confident mother, and her children sense that. She finds happiness in her work, her two children, in me. And she has done everything she wants to do – no matter how hard or impossible it has been. She truly is amazing.

A NOTE ON THE AUTHOR AND THE CO-AUTHOR

Kareena Kapoor Khan is one of India's best-known actresses. She is the mother of two boys.

Aditi Shah Bhimjyani is a freelance writer whose work has appeared in several publications. She lives in Mumbai with her family.

Scan the QR code with a QR scanner app or
type the link www.amazon.in/KareenaBabyList
on your internet browser to explore Kareena's
shopping list exclusively on Amazon.in

Shop for your baby's essentials at
www.amazon.in/baby

Ease your parenting journey with
Amazon Family by visiting
www.amazon.in/family

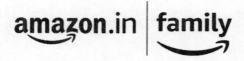

Click the QR Code with a QR scanner app or type the link into the Internet browser on your phone to download the Juggernaut app.

For our complete catalogue, visit www.juggernaut.in
To submit your book, send a synopsis and two sample chapters to books@juggernaut.in
For all other queries, write to contact@juggernaut.in